The Scientific Basis of Drug Therapy
in Psychiatry

THE SCIENTIFIC BASIS OF
DRUG THERAPY
IN
PSYCHIATRY

THE SCIENTIFIC BASIS OF
DRUG THERAPY
IN
PSYCHIATRY

A Symposium at
St. Bartholomew's Hospital, London
7th and 8th September, 1964

Edited by

JOHN MARKS

and

C. M. B. PARE

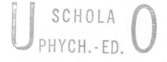

SYMPOSIUM PUBLICATIONS DIVISION
PERGAMON PRESS
OXFORD · [LONDON] · EDINBURGH · NEW YORK
PARIS · FRANKFURT

Pergamon Press Ltd., Headington Hill Hall, Oxford
4 & 5 Fitzroy Square, London W.1

Pergamon Press (Scotland) Ltd., 2 & 3 Teviot Place, Edinburgh 1

Pergamon Press Inc., 122 East 55th St., New York 10022

Pergamon Press GmbH, Kaiserstrasse 75, Frankfurt-am-Main

First edition 1965
Reprinted 1965

Library of Congress Catalog Card No. 65-16261

PRINTED IN GREAT BRITAIN BY BELL AND BAIN LIMITED, GLASGOW
(2257/65)

EDITORS' NOTE

IN order to achieve rapid publication the editors have not sent the proofs to the authors, and accept responsibility for any mistakes.

The editors acknowledge their gratitude to Mr. W. E. Harding and Mrs. Harrison in the preparation of this book.

Financial help in the organization of the symposium was given by Roche Products.

J.M.
C.M.B.P.

December 1964

CONTENTS

PAGE

List of participants   ix

Introduction   xiii

SESSION I

Basic concepts

Anatomy and physiology of the emotions and their relation to psycho-active drugs—H. E. HIMWICH   3

Methods of assessment of psychological effects of drugs in animals—HANNAH STEINBERG   25

Methods of assessment of psychological effects of drugs in man—M. HAMILTON   39

Invited discussants

    A. SUMMERFIELD   44

    I. OSWALD   46

General discussion   50

SESSION II

Major tranquillizers

Clinical use of the phenothiazines—J. DENHAM   55

Mode of action of the phenothiazines—D. RICHTER   63

Structure functional relationships within the phenothiazine class—P. SAINSBURY   71

Use of other drugs in the treatment of the schizophrenic—W. H. TRETHOWAN   79

Invited discussants

    J. R. SMYTHIES   90

    K. RAWNSLEY   93

General discussion   96

SESSION III

Antidepressants

Some clinical aspects of antidepressant drugs—C. M. B. PARE   103

Pharmacology of monoamine oxidase inhibitors—A. PLETSCHER   115

Some ideas on the mode of action of imipramine-type antidepressants
—B. B. BRODIE   127

Invited discussants

  A. C. TAIT   147

  P. J. DALLY   149

General discussion   152

SESSION IV

Anti-anxiety compounds

Use of drugs in anxiety states—F. A. JENNER   157

Mode of action of anti-anxiety compounds—G. A. HEISE   165

Invited discussants

  M. A. PARTRIDGE   179

  E. B. DAVIES   181

General discussion   185

SESSION V

General considerations

Interactions involving drugs used in psychiatry—J. MARKS   191

General discussion   202

Drug therapy in perspective—L. REES   205

Designation of compounds and their chemical and trade names   207

Index   211

LIST OF PARTICIPANTS

Chairmen

LINFORD REES, Esq., M.D., F.R.C.P., D.P.M.,
Saint Bartholomew's Hospital,
London, E.C.1.

Professor W. M. MILLAR, M.D., F.R.C.P.,
Department of Mental Health,
The University of Aberdeen,
Aberdeen.

Professor Sir AUBREY LEWIS, M.D., F.R.C.P.,
The Maudsley Hospital,
Denmark Hill, London, S.E.5.

WILLIAM SARGANT, Esq., M.A., F.R.C.P., D.P.M.,
St. Thomas's Hospital,
Westminster Bridge, London, S.E.1.

Speakers

BERNARD B. BRODIE, Esq., Ph.D.,
National Heart Institute,
National Institutes of Health,
Bethesda, Md., U.S.A.

P. J. DALLY, Esq., M.B., B.S., M.R.C.P., D.P.M.,
The Westminster Hospital,
Horseferry Road,
Westminster, London, S.W.1.

E. BERESFORD DAVIES, Esq., M.A., M.D., D.P.M.,
The United Cambridge Hospitals,
Trumpington Street, Cambridge.

JOHN DENHAM, Esq., M.D., L.R.C.P., M.R.C.S., D.P.M..
Long Grove Hospital,
Epsom, Surrey.

Professor MAX HAMILTON, M.D., D.P.M.,
Department of Psychiatry,
The University of Leeds, Leeds, 1.

ix

GEORGE A. HEISE, Esq., M.D.,
Associate Professor of Psychology,
Indiana University,
Bloomington, Indiana, U.S.A.

HAROLD E. HIMWICH, Esq., M.D.,
Director, Research Division, Department of Mental Health,
Galesburg State Research Hospital,
Galesburg, Illinois, U.S.A.

F. A. JENNER, Esq., Ph.D., M.B., Ch.B., D.P.M.,
Medical Research Council Unit,
Hollymoor Hospital,
Northfield, Birmingham.

J. MARKS, Esq., M.A., M.D., M.R.C.P.,
Downing College, Cambridge.

IAN OSWALD, Esq., M.A., M.D., D.SC., D.P.M.,
Department of Psychological Medicine,
The University of Edinburgh,
Edinburgh, 8.

C. M. B. PARE, Esq., M.D., M.R.C.P., D.P.M.,
Saint Bartholomew's Hospital,
London, E.C.1.

M. A. PARTRIDGE, Esq., M.A., D.M., M.R.C.P., L.M.S.S.A., D.P.M.,
St. George's Hospital,
Hyde Park Corner, London, S.W.1.

Professor A. PLETSCHER, M.D.,
Director, Medical Research Department,
F. Hoffmann–La Roche & Co., Basle, Switzerland.

Professor Kenneth Rawnsley, M.B., M.R.C.P., D.P.M.,
Department of Psychiatry,
The University of Cardiff, Cardiff.

DEREK RICHTER, Esq., M.A., Ph.D., M.R.C.S., L.R.C.P.,
Medical Research Council Neuropsychiatric Unit,
Carshalton, Surrey.

P. SAINSBURY, Esq., B.A., M.D., D.P.M.,
Medical Research Council Clinic,
Psychiatric Research Group,
Graylingwell Hospital, Chichester, Sussex.

J. R. SMYTHIES, Esq., M.A., M.D., M.R.C.P., D.P.M.,
Department of Psychological Medicine,
The University of Edinburgh,
Edinburgh, 8.

HANNAH STEINBERG, Ph.D.,
Department of Pharmacology,
University College,
Gower Street, London, W.C.1.

Professor A. SUMMERFIELD, Ph.D.,
Department of Psychology,
Birkbeck College, University of London,
London, W.C.1.

A. C. TAIT, Esq., M.B., Ch.B., D.P.H., D.P.M.,
Director of Clinical Research,
Crichton Royal Hospital, Dumfries.

Professor W. H. TRETHOWAN, F.R.A.C.P., F.R.C.P., D.P.M.,
Department of Psychiatry,
The University of Birmingham,
Edgbaston, Birmingham, 15.

INTRODUCTION

LINFORD REES

LADIES and gentlemen, I extend to you a warm welcome to St. Bartholomew's Hospital. The hospital has a long history. It was first established in 1125 and has occupied the same site ever since. Among the many illustrious physicians to work at St. Bartholomew's was William Harvey the discoverer of the circulation of the blood and the first person to apply the scientific method in clinical research. It is appropriate that a hospital with such a long history should be associated with a Symposium on one of the most recent and rapidly developing fields in medicine. In just over a decade psychotropic drugs have had a great impact on psychiatric practice and stimulated an immense amount of research.

The aim of this Symposium is to review the present state of knowledge of the clinical and therapeutic effects and the mode of action of the various psychotropic drugs. We are fortunate in having many leading authorities to speak to us on their special field of research.

It will be as important for future research for us to know about the difficulties and problems outstanding as well as the scientifically established advances in this advancing and important part of medicine.

I would like to thank the speakers, discussants, Chairmen, and all participants in the Symposium, and also to express our appreciation for the valuable support given by Roche Products.

SESSION I
BASIC CONCEPTS
Chairman: LINFORD REES

ANATOMY AND PHYSIOLOGY OF THE EMOTIONS AND THEIR RELATION TO PSYCHOACTIVE DRUGS

HAROLD E. HIMWICH

Summary—During recent years, methods have been devised for measuring certain types of brain activity and such information has made it possible to speculate in some detail on the physiological substrates of emotional activity. The first part of this paper reviews such information including recent advances in neuroanatomy and neurochemistry. In the second part the suggested site of action of some recently discovered groups of drugs and relationships between pharmacological findings and clinical effects are discussed.

Résumé—Pendant ces dernières années, des méthodes ont ètè mises au point pour mesurer certains genres d'activité cérébrale et une telle information a rendu possible d'avancer des hypothèses détaillées sur les substrats physiologiques de l'activité émotionnelle. La première partie de cette communication est consacrée à une telle information et inclut les progrès récents faits dans la neuro-anatomie et la neuro-chimie. Dans la seconde partie, on discute du point d'impact présumé de certains groupes de substances découverts récemment et des rapports entre les données pharmacologiques et les effets cliniques.

Zusammenfussung—In den letzten Jahren sind Methoden zur Messung bestimmter Arten zentralnervöser Aktivität entwickelt worden, und mit den dadurch erlangten Kenntnissen ist es möglich geworden, ziemlich differenzierte Spekulationen über die physiologischen Substrate emotioneller Funktionen anzustellen. Im ersten Teil des Vortrags wird ein Überblick über diese Kenntnisse und über die neuesten neuro-anatomischen und neurochemischen Forschungsergebnisse gegeben. Im zweiten Teil werden der hypothetische Angriffspunkt einiger in jüngster Zeit entdeckter Medikamentengruppen und die Beziehungen zwischen pharmakologischen Befunden und klinischen Effekten diskutiert.

WE have previously presented a concept of the neuroanatomical basis for the emotions. [1] In that formulation we reviewed the anatomical substrate of the emotions and included suggestions on the sites of action in the brain of chlorpromazine, reserpine and meprobamate. These three drugs were chosen as representatives of the phenothiazines, *Rauwolfia* alkaloids and substituted propanediols respectively and anatomical loci sensitive to their actions were compared with those of the sedative-hypnotic barbiturates. Advancing research, both basic and clinical, has however modified our viewpoints somewhat; not only our ideas of the functional organization of the reticular formation but also of the pharmacological responses to these drugs. Thus today we have a deeper understanding of the well-known group of

3

phenothiazine drugs. Moreover, relatively newer psychoactive agents have been developed: imipramine and other members of this antidepressant group of drugs for the treatment of the endogenous depressions as well as the monoamine oxidase inhibitors, of which iproniazid is the prototype, help in the management of atypical depressions. In addition the anti-anxiety drug chlordiazepoxide has come to the fore. These newer psychoactive agents will also be considered within the co-ordinates of the anatomical, physiological and pharmacological analysis of their influences on the brain. It is advisable to use the term neuropharmacological when the most apparent action of a drug is on neurological structures, an example of which would be the anti-parkinson drugs, and psychopharmacological where a drug is administered, for example, to allay anxiety or ameliorate psychotic symptoms, but this dichotomous use of the two terms is only a pragmatic device. We would not care to separate the brain and the mind from each other in the conception we are about to describe. Moreover, relations have been uncovered between the extrapyramidal apparatus and mental symptoms.[2, 3] To describe this global action we employ the rather clumsy term neuropsychopharmacology which has come into general use.

PART I: NEUROANATOMICAL BASIS OF THE EMOTIONS

In opening the discussion on the neuroanatomical and neurophysiological basis for the emotions, we shall begin with the concept that the brain acts as a unit. The brain is formed of a bundle of structures representing different potentialities and different activities, but we find a great unifying mechanism in reverberating circuits, as the brain parts are interconnected by neural pathways which serve to complete reverberating circuits. A unified action of the brain, therefore, is attained by the interactions of these various structures which can partly explain why, for example, an emotional arousal caused by an unpleasant experience does not cease the moment the stimulus is over, as on the contrary we continue to glower and smoulder for a long time afterwards as the positive feedbacks continue to reverberate. Such continued processes may lead to psychopathology for example to pathological anxiety. But we have both positive feedbacks and negative ones, and the latter function more frequently. Thus inhibitions and brakes are applied by the various components of the reverberating circuits and the total response of the body frequently ceases with the cessation of the application of the stimulus. The first brilliant suggestion for the function of a reverberating circuit in explaining emotional experience came from Papez in 1937.[4] He said, " Is emotion a magic product or is it a physiological process which depends on an anatomical mechanism. . . . It is proposed that the hypothalamus, the anterior thalamic nuclei, the gyrus cingulae, the hippocampus and their interconnections constitute a harmonious mechanism which may elaborate the functions of central emotion as well as participate in emotional expression " (Fig. 1). This fertile suggestion achieves its merit by combining in an anatomic and functional formulation the chief centre for the co-ordination of emotional behaviour, namely the hypothalamus with a portion of the neocortex, the cingulate gyrus, thus bringing a component of discrete awareness to the more vague but nevertheless powerful impulses which are regulated by the older cortical areas. The structures of the Papez circuit

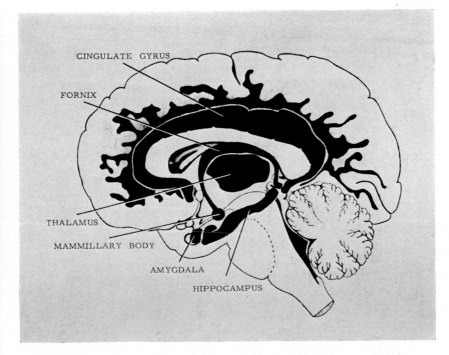

FIG. 1. Papez circuit. On stimulation of the hippocampus this structure relays impulses via the fornix to the mammillary bodies of the hypothalamus. From that area they continue to the anterior thalamic nuclei and to the cingulate gyrus of the cerebral cortex. The functional circuit is completed by fibres leaving the cingulate gyrus by way of the cingulum and returning to the hippocampus via the hippo-campal gyrus.[15]

and some other phylogenetically ancient cortical structures are included in the term limbic system and we shall see that the regulation of hypothalamic mechanisms is effected by the other members of the limbic system which apply either positive or negative controls, i.e. positive or negative feedbacks. The central position of the hypothalamus in emotions depends upon its function as the chief outlet for the neural messages chiefly from primitive parts of the brain to effector organs, striated muscle, smooth muscle and glands[5] and this central control is advantageous for example in providing

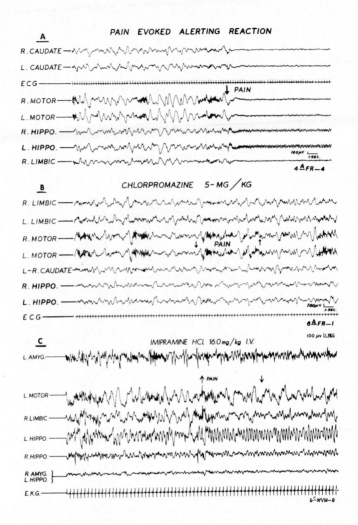

FIG. 2. Alert EEG patterns evoked by pain and prevented by chlorpromazine and imipramine. (A) Bilateral leads are taken from various cerebral structures as indicated: on left side, electroencephalographic control pattern of resting rabbit; on right side, the effect of pinching rabbit's leg. (B) Change produced by chlorpromazine (5 mg/kg) in electroencephalographic pattern in response to pain. Note the absence of the alerting reaction to pain.[27] (C) Effects of imipramine HCl on EEG arousal following peripheral pain stimulation. Note that the EEG arousal response to pain stimulation is blocked after the administration of imipramine HCl, 16 mg/kg (Himwich, H. E. Similarities between tranquillizers and antidepressants. Memorial Research Monographs Naka. Committee on Celebration of 60th Birthday of Prof. S. Naka, Osaka, Japan, pp. 125–142, (1960).

visceral support for the great expenditures of energy involved in the behavioural adaptations to emergency situations. But whether or not appreciation of emotional feeling occurs in the hypothalamus is doubtful.[6] Rather
discriminative awareness of the emotions probably requires the active
participation of the thalamus in a rudimentary way and of neocortical areas
in a more discriminatory manner by means of reverberating circuits like that
of Papez.[5]

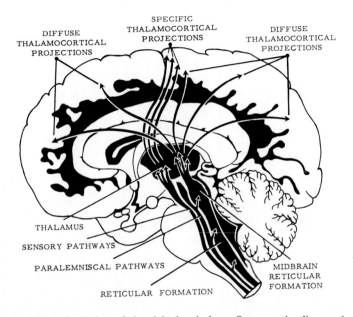

FIG. 3. Mid-sagittal view of the right hemisphere. Sensory stimuli ascend the
lemniscal classical sensory pathways and stimulate the specific sensory nuclei of
the thalamus whence impulses are transmitted to the cortical specific somato-
sensory areas via the specific thalamocortical projections. The ascending
functions of the mesodiencephalic activating system may be said to start with
impulses in collaterals from the paralemniscal sensory pathways to the reticular
formation which is thus aroused and sends signals to the unspecific thalamic
nuclei where the diffuse thalamocortical projections to the cortex take their
origin.[1]

One of the oldest parts of the brain involved in behaviour, the reticula
formation, is well developed even in amphibia[7] and continues to exert
important influences even in mammals. This polysynaptic structure is
situated centrally in the lower brainstem with an important representation
in the midbrain and extends rostrally to the hypothalamus, subthalamus and
thalamus to affect behaviour in a complex fashion. Some reticular impulses
are transmitted directly to the neocortex. Others go first to the unspecific
thalamic nuclei which in turn relay the messages diffusely to the neocortex.

The midbrain reticular formation and the thalamic projections may act in conjunction with each other and together they are responsible for the arousal reaction of the EEG (Fig. 2A). The combined activity of these two structures is recognized in the term mesodiencephalic activating system

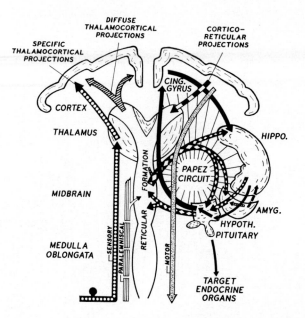

FIG. 4. Diagrammatic transverse section of brain. The left half of the figure portrays lemniscal sensory pathways to the specific sensory nuclei and the specific sensory areas of the cortex (white dots on black arrows) as well as paralemniscal ones (black and white vertical stripes) and collaterals (black and white arrow) to the reticular formation (white) which in turn relays impulses to the cortex via the diffuse thalamocortical projections (shaded). On the right side of the figure a feedback from the cortex in the cortico-reticular projections completes a reverberating circuit between the cortex and the reticular formation. The Papez circuit (in black) is portrayed connecting the hippocampus, hypothalamus (mammillary body), (anterior thalamic nuclei are not represented), cingulate gyrus and returning to the hippocampus. The connections of the Papez circuit with the amygdala and reticular formation are indicated by arrows containing white diamond shapes. Fibres originating in the nuclei of Gudden and Bechterow, situated in the reticular formation, pass directly to the hypothalamus, to the septal area (not indicated) and to the hippocampus and amygdala. These structures send impulses to the reticular formation to complete reverberating circuits. These areas represent a portion of the anatomical substrate of behavioural adjustments occurring especially with strong stimulation of the organism. The motor pathways from the cortex to the spinal cord (stipled arrow) are included in the right half of the diagram. The reticular formation also possesses important descending motor activities including extrapyramidal regulation. (This figure is adapted from Galambos[7] in paper by Himwich, H. E., Functional organization of the brain, past and present. *J. Nerv. Ment. Dis.* **130**, 505–519, 1960.)

(MDAS)[8] and their respective physiologies have been worked out by Moruzzi and Magoun[9] as well as Jasper.[10] When we receive any kind of stimulus produced by sound, touch or pain, impulses are initiated which travel in sensory tracts and lemnisci to attain the sensory cortex by way of the specific thalamocortical fibres, thus bringing discrete information in regard to the character of the stimulus and its localization (Figs. 3 and 4). Simultaneously there are changes in the spontaneous EEG which loses its resting characteristics and assumes the alert pattern (Fig. 2A). It has been suggested that this change in the EEG is associated with the affect,[8] the emotional cloak accompanying sensory information, for example, accompanying a painful stimulus. Both the EEG and emotional reactions are maintained in part by a positive feedback mechanism formed by the corticopetal pathways, just described, and corticofugal fibres to the reticular formation, the cortico-reticular paths and together form another one of the reverberating circuits between the more primitive brain areas and the areas concerned most closely with discriminatory functions (Fig. 4). The EEG and emotional components of arousal are associated in addition with behavioural aspects as adjustments are made to the stimulus, for example, as the eyes turn to the site of stimulation and other appropriate changes in body posture are effected. Such adaptations are accomplished by impulses transmitted from the midbrain reticular formation to the hypothalamus which in turn co-ordinates the behavioural responses to the stimulus. Thus the midbrain reticular formation gives rise to impulses which are transmitted to various supra-reticular areas, to the neocortex and to the diffuse thalamic nuclei as well as the hypothalamus. The neocortical areas which are most intimately connected with the hypothalamic functions are the cingulate gyrus as well as the orbital surfaces of the frontal lobes for they also exert strong influences on the hypothalamus.[11] Far more powerful, however, than neocortical connections are those between the hypothalamus and other limbic structures.

Impulses making for arousal are accounted for in two ways. A prevalent viewpoint describes sensory impulses coursing centrally in the lemniscus and some of them attaining the reticular formation via lemniscal collaterals.[12] More recently Lindsley and Adey[13] as well as Morillo and Baylor[14] failed to find functional participation of lemniscal fibres in the arousal reaction and the latter investigators suggest that paralemniscal sensory paths, the spinoreticular, spinotectal and Lissauer's tracts provide the input to the reticular formation (Figs. 3 and 4). It should be emphasized that both viewpoints agree on the close relationship between discrete sensory awareness of a stimulus and EEG alerting and disagree only on the path by which the impulses making for EEG arousal arrive at the reticular formation.

The phylogenetically older portions of the cortex, associated with smell, are deeply involved in the regulation of emotional behaviour, as they bring

their influences to bear on hypothalamic mechanisms. Indeed the relationship between odours and the emotions are well known, and taking an example
from psychopathology, we note that schizophrenic patients with olfactory
hallucinations may present episodes of virulent exacerbations of symptoms.
One instance is afforded by a schizophrenic patient who brutally murdered

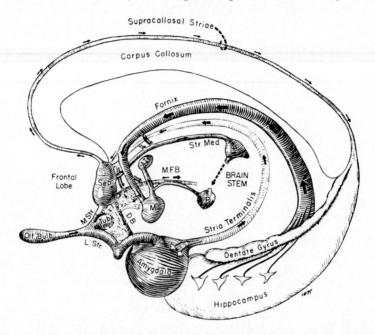

FIG. 5. Schematic representation of impulses from the olfactory bulb to the
septum, olfactory tubercle and amygdala. Impulses leave the amygdala via the
stria terminalis to attain the mammillary bodies of the hypothalamus, the septum
and midbrain. Another polysynaptic pathway is operative from the amygdala to
the hippocampus via the pyriform cortex, and there are also many other pathways
between the amygdala and hippocampus not indicated in the figure. A.T.—
anterior nucleus of the thalamus, D.B.—diagonal band of Broca, H.—habenula,
I.P.—interpenduncular nucleus, L. Str.—lateral olfactory stria, M.—mammillary
body, M.F.B.—medial forebrain bundle, M. Str.—medial olfactory stria, Olf.
Bulb—olfactory bulb, Sep.—region of the septal nuclei, Str. Med.—stria medul-
laria, Tub.—olfactory tubercle (head of the caudate immediately underneath).[15]

his two teen-age daughters. He said he had to do so because of the " smell
of death ". The olfactory bulb sends impulses to the septal olfactory tubercle
and amygdala and these structures pass them on to the hypothalamus[15]
(Fig. 5). Moreover, the amygdaloid nuclei are also in communication with
the hypothalamus via the stria terminalis (Fig. 4). Amygdaloid messages
attain the hippocampus partially by way of the uncus or pyriform cortex.[16]
Two-way communication between the amygdala and hippocampus also takes

place by means of numerous subcortical pathways.[17] The reticular formation sends afferents to the hypothalamus in a variety of ways; by connections to the olfactory tubercles and also by fibres originating in the nuclei of Gudden and Bechterev (Fig. 4) and hypothalamic feedbacks in turn transmit impulses to the reticular formation[18] to form a reverberating circuit that may evoke or maintain the arousal reaction. Thus by many pathways the hypothalamus is in connection with the septum, amygdala, hippocampus and the reticular formation and in this manner they affect the behavioural expressions regulated by the hypothalamus.

It is interesting to attempt to allocate the characteristic effects of the various component structures of the limbic system. In this regard we must refer to the pathfinding experiments of Klüver and Bucy on monkeys (*Macacus rhesus*).[19] These investigators removed the temporal lobes containing the amygdala and anterior hippocampus as well as the overlying uncus or pyriform cortex and noted that wild monkeys became tame. But today we might call them tranquillized. Stimuli previously capable of evoking signs of fear or rage were rendered innocuous by extirpation of these structures. Profound changes in behaviour were observed, for the strong motor and vocal reactions generally associated with anger or fear were no longer exhibited. There also were disturbances in the sexual sphere as the operated male primates became hypersexed. They copulated continuously for $\frac{1}{2}$ hour at a time, copulations that were often repeated again and again in a single day. In regard to the behavioural alterations of fear and rage, other workers have also reported that bilateral removal of the amygdala and hippocampus leads to placidity and emotional unresponsiveness.[20, 21, 22] Similarly extirpation of the orbital surface of the frontal lobe renders primates docile and devoid of fear.[11] In contrast to the above results lesions limited to the septal areas produce rage.[23] If we may regard the effects of extirpations as results of the loss of functional regulation exhibited by each of the parts, one may conclude that the amygdala and hippocampus as well as the orbital surface of the frontal lobe tend to increase emotional reactions while the septum depresses such expressions. MacLean[24] makes the additional points that the septum, hippocampus and cingulate gyrus are concerned with the preservation of the species, while in contrast the processes of obtaining food and the accompanying behavioural reactions, namely attack and defence, are more directly the concern of the frontotemporal portion of the limbic system including the amygdala and related structures. But he also emphasizes that there are strong connections between the two groups of structures as well as their integrated reactions.[24]

It is of more than passing interest that certain brain neurohormones including noradrenaline and serotonin occur in greatest concentrations in the phylogenetically older structures involved in the emotions but that neocortical areas are practically devoid of them (Fig. 6). The hypothalamus, for example, has a greater concentration of noradrenaline then any other brain area. Far behind are the structures next richest in noradrenaline including the septum and amygdaloid nuclei, the mesencephalic red nucleus and substantia nigra as well as the rhombencephalic reticular formation. Serotonin distribution is similar to that of noradrenaline except that the

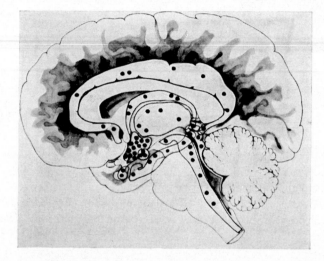

FIG. 6. Mid-sagittal view of the right hemisphere illustrating sites of brain neuro-hormones and especially those of serotonin and noradrenaline. The relative concentrations of neurohormones in the various brain areas are indicated by the number of filled circles within each area.[1]

preponderant position of noradrenaline in the hypothalamus is not duplicated and in addition serotonin is relatively more concentrated than noradrenaline in the caudate nucleus, putamen, globus pallidus and substantia nigra. Dopamine, closely related biochemically to noradrenaline and adrenaline, is found chiefly in the extrapyramidal system as it occurs in greatest amounts in the caudate nucleus and the putamen and is also well represented in the substantia nigra.[25]

PART II: SITES OF ACTION OF PSYCHOPHARMACOLOGICAL DRUGS IN RELATION TO THE STRUCTURE OF THE LIMBIC SYSTEM.

Because every drug affects to a greater or lesser degree all bodily and brain components it would be surprising if the psychoactive agents did not have many actions throughout the body, but as it turns out, the brain and particularly the limbic system present sites exquisitely sensitive to these drugs. Usually several limbic structures react and in a variety of ways. Thus the emotional components of behaviour are influenced most deeply by this group of drugs. Our analysis of the areas sensitive to psychoactive drugs will be made on the basis of animal experimentation, though differences of species are important considerations. Unfortunately it is more difficult to place deep electrodes in the human limbic system and to study limbic neurohormones in man than in animals. We do not suggest that the brain changes disclosed in animals can necessarily be interpreted in such a way that they have significance in relation to behavioural alterations of patients. We shall, however, point out correlations between the specific effects of psychoactive drugs on the animal brain and on the broader clinical changes whether or not, for example, the two different parameters both indicate tendencies toward tranquillization. In order to confine my observations to reasonable limits, only some findings in animals will be presented. Moreover, because of feedback mechanisms, it is difficult to know whether the observed results are primary or secondary especially when drug-induced changes appear spontaneously. When, however, a brain part is stimulated directly, for example by an electric current, the observed result, in the stimulated site, is more likely to be primary by nature.

Reserpine. The first drug we shall consider is reserpine, one of the two original tranquillizers, and now to a great extent replaced by the phenothiazines. Reserpine requires a longer period of time than the phenothiazines to build up its maximum tranquillizing effects. Moreover, when reserpine is first administered it may produce a period of worsening in the psychotic symptoms usually more marked and longer acting than those evoked by phenothiazine derivatives. In regard to the reticular formation, we formerly believed that the primary effect of reserpine was that of alerting[26, 27] but further experimentation has revealed that these activating effects come early and correlate with the early worsening actions of reserpine on behaviour (Fig. 7A). But once these initial reactions are completed we find that a sleep pattern is the chief characteristic of reserpine administration[28, 29] (Fig. 7B).

It is well known that reserpine releases brain neurohormones from their depots. The alert pattern occurs simultaneously with the increased amounts of free serotonin and noradrenaline as the neurohormonal stores are in process of depletion, but after this depletion is completed, and the neurohormonal levels are lowered, the spontaneous EEG assumes the resting pattern, frequently a sign of sedation in animals and of tranquillization in patients. With such a drug-induced type of EEG, sensory stimuli fail to evoke the EEG arousal and probably the associated emotional response is also diminished in intensity.[26, 27]

The actions of reserpine on hypothalamic mechanisms are complex. It is true that noradrenergic ones are prevented but those of the cholinergic type are augmented, as seen for example in the constriction of the pupil and by the bradycardia. Perhaps another reason why reserpine is not as satisfactory clinically as the phenothiazines[30] is seen in its stimulating influence on limbic structures which may exhibit spontaneous seizures with reserpine.[31] The total effect of any medicament on behaviour depends, of course, on the summation of all its influences on the brain, and with reserpine, the resultant is less influential in the direction of tranquillization than with the phenothiazines.

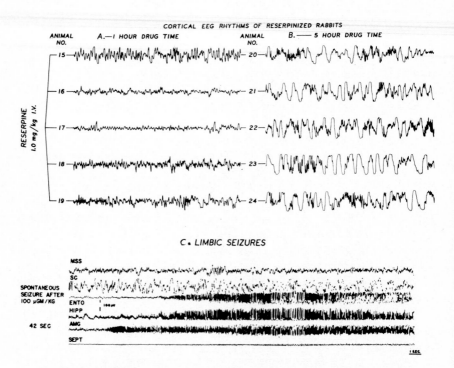

FIG. 7. Cortical EEG tracings from 13 animals injected with reserpine (1·0 mg/kg) before surgical preparation. Note the presence of EEG activation at 1 hr (A) and its absence at 5 hr (B).[27] Electroencephalographic tracings recorded following administration of 0·1 mg/kg of reserpine (C). Note spontaneous seizures of limbic structures. Recording leads are as follows: MSS, median suprasylvian gyrus; SC, sensory cortex; ENTO, entorhinal cortex; HIPP, hippocampus; AMG, amygdala; SEPT, septum.[31]

Phenothiazines. The phenothiazine derivatives constitute the largest group of psychoactive drugs. From the clinical viewpoint there are important quantitative differences between their actions, but the qualitative similarities of the various phenothiazines facilitate their discussion as a group. Some important phenothiazine derivatives are chlorpromazine, triflupromazine, promazine, methoxypromazine, mepazine, piperacetazine, prochlorperazine, perphenazine, trifluoperazine, fluphenazine, acetophenazine and carphenazine. In an analysis of their sites of action, we will consider first the MDAS including its caudal and rostral components, the reticular formation and the diffuse thalamocortical projections. It is true that the MDAS as a whole is cholinergic in function and atropine for example can block EEG arousal caused by practically any kind of stimulus. These inhibiting effects of atropine occur because the rostral component of the MDAS is cholinergic, the component which determines the character of the EEG whether it is resting or aroused (Fig. 2A). On the other hand, the caudal constituent, the reticular component, responds to adrenergic stimuli, probably not by a direct action[31] but due to the effects of adrenaline and adrenaline-like substance on afferent collaterals to the reticular formation.[32] The blocking effect of phenothiazines on the EEG is in accordance with their cholinolytic action[34, 35] even though it is much weaker than that of atropine. Figure 2B presents an example of the failure of EEG arousal due to the inhibiting action of chlorpromazine. Whatever the exact mechanism for this inhibition, there is no doubt that the EEG alerting responses to a painful stimulus do not occur under chlorpromazine and that the usual accompanying disturbing affect is also ameliorated. It is well known that patients bear pain with less difficulty under phenothiazine therapy than without one of these drugs.[27] Phenothiazine tranquillization also correlates with depression of the hypothalamus and reticular formation, areas containing relatively high concentrations of the neurohormones, and neurohormonal actions are inhibited by this group of drugs.[34] As the blood-brain barrier is permeable to the phenothiazines, there is no reason to doubt that they penetrate the hypothalamus, and in addition it has been found that the phenothiazines reduce to some degree excitability of the extra-hypothalamic limbic structures as well. [31] The tranquillization produced by the phenothiazines would seem to be associated with both direct and indirect influences on the hypothalamus. We should like to emphasize that such tranquillization is not specific as it is exhibited irrespective of the diagnostic category of the patient.

It is another question entirely to explain the specific antipsychotic powers by which hallucinations and delusions of schizophrenic patients are mitigated or eliminated by the phenothiazines. Perhaps here the dampening of neurocortical components of arousal and the maintenance of the resting EEG patterns despite disturbing stimuli should be mentioned. In any case because false sensory interpretations and unrealistic thinking in schizophrenic patients are ameliorated by the phenothiazines, their therapeutic actions would seem necessarily to involve neocortical functions. For that reason we suggest that by virtue of the Papez and similar reverberating circuits which involve neocortical areas, the effects of the phenothiazines on the older brain parts are indirectly brought to bear on those functions which are allocated in large part to the neocortex. Thus far we have mentioned possible mechanisms for tranquillization and antipsychotic powers. A third psychotherapeutic advantage of the phenothiazines is found in the clinical improvements observed in some depressed patients treated with the phenothiazines,[37] and this aspect will be considered in the next section on the antidepressant drugs.

Drugs used in the treatment of patients with depressive moods. One group of antidepressant drugs is employed in the management of psychotic depression of endogenous origin; melancholia and the depressive phase of the manic depressive psychosis. Previous to these antidepressants, endogenous depressions were treated best with electroconvulsive therapy. This group of drugs was initiated with the advent of imipramine and soon included amitriptyline and subsequently desmethylimipramine and two somewhat different chemical forms of desmethylamitriptyline as well as opipramol. We should point out that this antidepressant action is specific against endogenous depressions and stimulating actions on behaviour of a non-depressed individual are neither as marked nor as constant.

Another group of antidepressant drugs secures improvements in the atypical depressions in which either anxiety or hysteroid features assume predominant positions in the clinical picture.[36] For these atypical depressions, however, we have another group of drugs, the monoamine oxidase inhibitors (MAOI), which started with iproniazid and now includes other irreversible inhibitors like phenelzine, nialamide, isocarboxazid as well as reversible ones like tranylcypromine. Their therapeutic actions can not be regarded as specific for they exert euphoriant effects in individuals who are not depressed. The side reactions of the monoamine oxidase inhibitors are more profound and frequent than those of the imipramine group, yet the untoward results can usually be prevented or managed should they arise. At this point the phenothiazines are also mentioned as advantageous in certain types of depression as indicated by a study in which patients were chosen not because their diagnosis fitted into any of the usually depressive syndromes but rather as having depression as major symptom. In addition they exhibited a large component of anxiety.[37]

The basic actions of the three groups of drugs, useful in the treatment of the various kinds of depressions, all have in common the ability to produce the stimulating effect of EEG alerting (Fig. 8A, B and C). But only the monoamine oxidase inhibitors as their name implies, inhibit monoamine oxidase, an enzyme concerned with the oxidation of serotonin and noradrenaline among other monoamines. As a result of this inhibition most members of this group of drugs increase the concentrations of serotonin and noradrenaline in the brain, an effect opposite to that of the tranquillizer, reserpine. What relationship there may be between the rise of the brain neurohormones and the behavioural improvement is still to be elucidated. But it is suggestive that the EEG arousal is associated with a rapid elevation of serotonin in the brainstem.[38] Noradrenaline rises too but more slowly.

The phenothiazine and imipramine groups share many actions. It has been shown, for example, that both groups affect the spontaneous EEG in a biphasic manner. Smaller doses induce the resting or sleeping patterns while larger ones cause EEG alerting.[28] These experiments were all made with

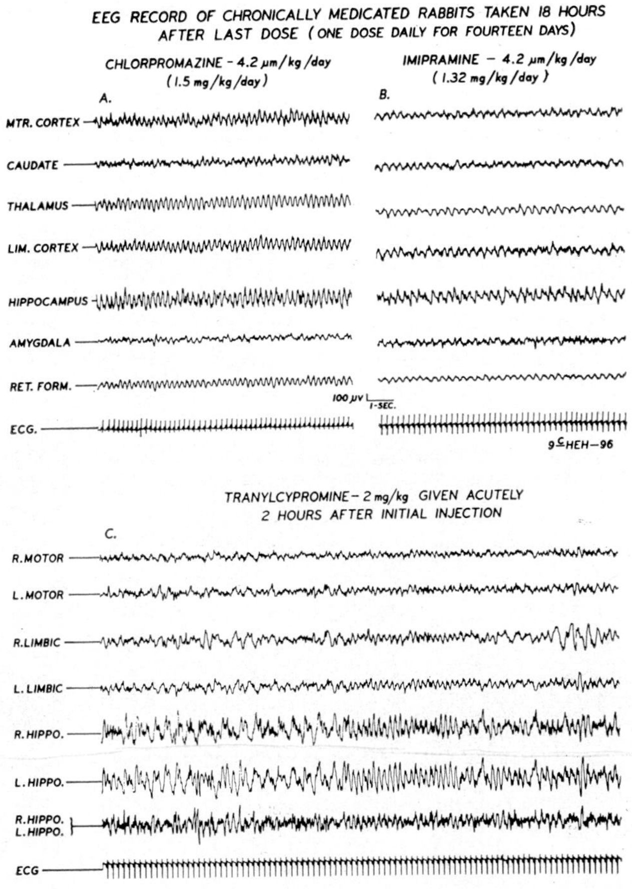

FIG. 8. Spontaneous EEG activation resulting from chronic medication with either chlorpromazine (A) imipramine[39] (B) or injections of tranylcypromine[38] (C).

acute dosages. But what may be more significant from the clinical viewpoint is observed with daily administration similar to that required in the treatment of patients. Small daily doses of either a phenothiazine or imipramine-like drug will change the spontaneous EEG from sleep to the arousal pattern.[35, 39] But in contrast to the phenothiazines, six of the seven antidepressants studied produced spike-like activity in subcortical structures, particularly the olfactory bulb (Fig. 9).[40] Thus not only clinically are there differences between the phenothiazines, the imipramine-like antidepressants, and MAO inhibitors, but our analysis also discloses that each of the three groups of drugs seems to act differently on the brain.

Finally it should be pointed out that just as thioridazine, a phenothiazine, possesses desirable clinical effects in patients with various types of de-

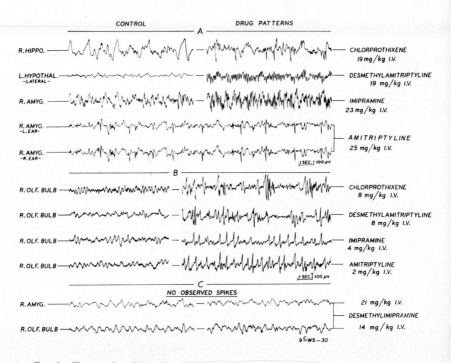

FIG. 9. Changes in rabbit EEG induced by antidepressant drugs devoid of monoamine oxidase inhibition. A: Frequently observed variations of spike-like EEG patterns of positive polarity (downward deflections) evoked by antidepressant drugs in three different cerebral areas. The last two tracings represent a special control recording of polarity of spikes as a function of ear reference. The spiking is drug-induced. B: Mixed patterns of negative (upward deflections) and biphasic polarity spike-like EEG patterns in olfactory bulb. C: Failure of the antidepressant, desmethylimipramine, to evoke either positive spikes in amygdala or negative spikes in olfactory bulb.[40]

pression,[37] so does imipramine produce tranquillization in patients with schizophrenia,[41] a change which correlates with an action of that drug to block neurohormonal actions, though it does so less effectively than chlorpromazine. Some of these patients with schizophrenic reactions treated with imipramine also suffered from superimposed depressions and therefore improvement in mood might have been expected. But others were without any signs of depression and nevertheless benefited from imipramine, exhibiting a desirable tranquillization. The point we would like to make is that though we frequently name drugs for some outstanding characteristic such as tranquillization or antidepressant activity, yet their psychopharmacological analysis discloses that they influence many sites of action in similar ways. The phenothiazines and the imipramine-like antidepressants particularly have actions in common. Perhaps that is one of the secrets of the clinical successes of the phenothiazines on one hand and the imipramine-like antidepressants on the other hand, for they both possess tranquillizing and antidepressant properties.

Drugs for the treatment of the milder neuroses. For the grave neuroses the same drugs are used as for patients with the psychoses but not for the same reason, for these drugs evoke the general action of tranquillization rather than specific effects. But in the milder forms of neuroses including patients with neurotic or reactive depressions the milder tranquillizers bring strong adjunctive support to psychotherapy. By diminishing anxiety and tension they help to tide over particularly bad periods characterized by disabling anxiety which may occur during the course of psychotherapy. Unlike the stronger tranquillizers, the milder ones exhibit their actions less widely on fewer brain regions. They are also less potent and accordingly exhibit fewer and milder side reactions.

Chlordiazepoxide. In usual doses chlordiazepoxide and the closely related diazepam possess valuable assets in the amelioration of anxiety whether or not associated with somatic complaints. These two drugs are an aid in the treatment of patients with depressed mood probably because the accompanying anxiety is alleviated. They exert only weak or no effects upon the neocortex, MDAS and neurohormonal depots but their clinical actions seem to correlate with their depressant influences on limbic structures, the septum, amygdala and hippocampus.[42] Such a depression may simulate to a certain degree the tranquillization observed with animals subjected to extirpations of these structures. Another example of this inhibiting action is seen on electrical stimulation of the amygdala when the resulting evoked potentials are recorded from the hippocampus. The administration of chlordiazepoxide or diazepam[15, 43, 44] reduces the hippocampal responses (Fig. 10B). As mentioned in the first section of this paper, the amygdala and hippocampus may exert facilitatory influences upon the hypothalamus and this reduction of the sensitivity may indirectly render hypothalamic mechanisms less susceptible to stimuli and therefore diminish reactions to stressful influences, thus ameliorating anxiety. Such a desirable clinical response also correlates with the ability of these drugs to inhibit, to a moderate degree, the alerting reaction to stimuli (Fig. 10A).[45]

Meprobamate. Meprobamate calms the tense, nervous depressed patient so frequently seen in general practice and is also used to allay anxiety

C

occurring with the exogenous or reactive depressions usually considered exogenous in origin and sometimes termed neurotic depressions. It is striking that in usual doses this drug does not influence significantly the discriminative functions of the neocortex nor those of either component of the MDAS to affect EEG patterns. Neurohormonal depots, moreover, are not altered.[46] On the other hand,[1] meprobamate exerts potent effects on some limbic structures. For in rats exhibiting irritability due to septal lesions[47] meprobamate sets aside their symptoms in a dramatic manner.

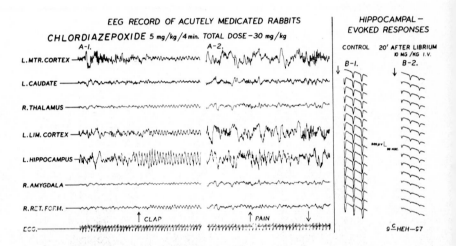

FIG. 10. Effects of chlordiazepoxide on spontaneous EEG recordings and evoked hippocampal responses following stimulation of the amygdala. A1: Control EEG revealing the change from a resting to an alerting pattern in response to a stimulus of hand clapping. A2: blocking by chlordiazepoxide of alerting due to pain.[45] B1: Hippocampal responses to single shocks and repetitive stimulation of lateral nucleus of the amygdala. B2: Response to repetitive stimulation 20 min after i.v. injection of 10 mg/kg of chlordiazepoxide. Note gradual impairment of evoked response.[43]

Similarly, meprobamate has been found effective in rendering the hippocampus less sensitive as the after-discharge following its electrical stimulation is first reduced and finally eliminated[48] (Fig. 11). This reduction of hippocampal activity is probably an indirect source of hypothalamic depression and may bring on an attendant diminution of anxiety.

Barbiturates. The barbiturates possess potent inhibiting influences on many brain structures. They depress significantly the MDAS due to a direct action upon its caudal component, namely the reticular formation. They, therefore, block both the EEG (Fig. 12A and B) and the behavioural elements of arousal, all of which are mediated by the midbrain reticular formation (see Part I of this paper, pp. 8–9). Thus behavioural responses to stimuli are diminished. The barbiturates moderately increase neurohormonal stores, an increase which however is secondary to central depression.[49] The barbiturates diminish directly the excitability of the hypothalamic functions[50] including the centre for wakefulness.[51] Moreover, the limbic

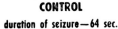

CONTROL

duration of seizure—64 sec.

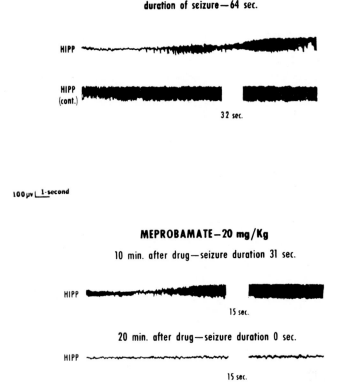

FIG. 11. The effect of meprobamate to shorten duration of after-discharge produced in the hippocampus by local electrical stimulation. Control record prior to drug administration is presented as well as records made 10 and 20 min after administration of meprobamate. Each tracing begins at end of stimulation period.[48]

structures feeding into the hypothalamus are rendered less sensitive to stimuli as shown by the Killams[30] (Fig. 12B). All these depressant actions present sources of the sedative-hypnotic powers of the barbiturates. Perhaps an even more significant difference between the tranquillizers in general and the barbiturates as a group is that the latter exert more profound effects on neocortical areas associated with the so-called higher functions of the mind. For that reason these drugs interfere with therapeutic processes which require

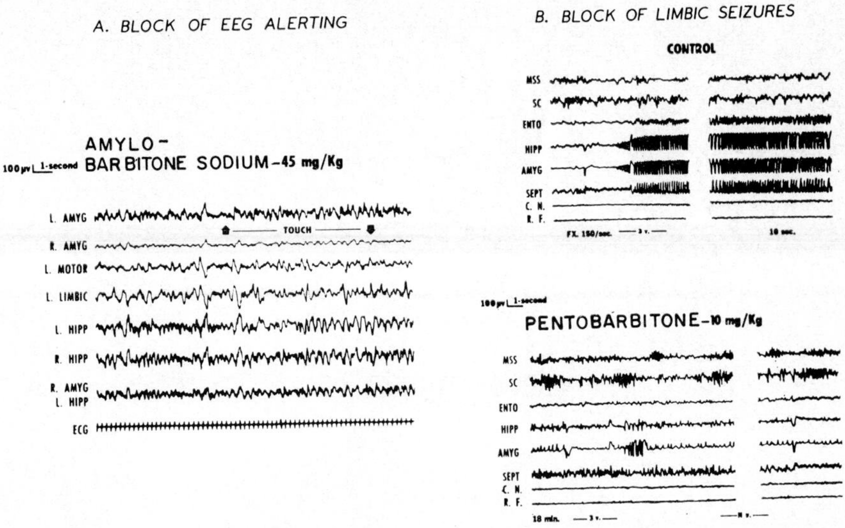

A. BLOCK OF EEG ALERTING   B. BLOCK OF LIMBIC SEIZURES

FIG. 12. A: EEG alerting in response to touch is entirely eliminated by amylobarbitone sodium as the reticular formation is inhibited.[1] B: Limbic lobe seizures resulting from stimulation of the fornix were eliminated by pentobarbitone.[31] The blocking action of pentobarbitone on seizures was confined to the limbic lobe. Recordings were taken from median suprasylvian (MSS), sensory cortex (SC), entorhinal cortex (ENTO), hippocampus (HIPP), amygdala (AMYG), septum (SEPT), caudate nucleus (C.N.) and reticular formation of the mesencephalon (R.F.).

TABLE 1. SUMMARY OF ACTIONS OF PSYCHOACTIVE DRUGS DISCUSSED IN THIS COMMUNICATION

Site of action	Reserpine	Phenothiazines	Imipramine-like anti-depressants	MAOI anti-depressants	Chlordiaz-epoxide	Meprobamate	Barbiturates
MDAS; EEG block or arousal	Early arousal. Later block	Acute block. Chronic arousal	Acute block. Chronic arousal	Arousal	Block	No effect	Block
Limbic structures	Stimulate	Inhibit	Stimulate	No effect	Inhibit	Inhibit	Inhibit
Neuro-hormones	Deplete	Block	Block	Increase	No effect	No effect	Increase
Neocortex	No effect	No effect	No effect	No effect	No effect	No effect	Depress
Respiratory centres	No effect	No effect	No effect	No effect	No effect	No effect	Depress

understanding and cooperation, especially with neurotic patients. In addition, in large doses they present a danger of respiratory failure. Thus in many ways tranquillizers are to be preferred over the barbiturates in the clinical management of patients with mental disorders. A summary of the salient actions of the principal psychoactive drugs is presented in Table 1.

REFERENCES

1. HIMWICH, H. E., *J. Neuropsychiat.* **3**, 279 (1962).
2. BRUNE, G. G., MORPURGO, C., BIELKUS, A., KOBAYASHI, T., TOURLENTES, T. T. and HIMWICH, H. E., *Comp. Psychiat.* **3**, 227 (1962).
3. BRUNE, G. G., KOBAYASHI, T., BULL, C., TOURLENTES, T. T. and HIMWICH, H. E., *Comp. Psychiat.* **3**, 292 (1962).
4. PAPEZ, J. W., *Arch. Neurol. Psychiat.* **38**, 725 (1937).
5. COBB, S., *Emotions and Clinical Medicine*, Norton, New York, 1960.
6. MASSERMAN, J. H., *Amer. J. Psychiat.* **98**, 633 (1942).
7. HERRICK, C. J., *The Brain of the Tiger Salamander*, University of Chicago Press, Chicago, 1948.
8. HIMWICH, H. E., *Science* **127**, 59 (1958).
9. MORUZZI, G., and MAGOUN, H. W., *Electroenceph. clin. Neurophysiol.* **1**, 455 (1949).
10. JASPER, H., *Electroenceph. clin. Neurophysiol.* **1**, 405 (1949).
11. FULTON, J., PRIBRAM, K. H., STEVENSON, J. A. F. and WALL, P. D., *Trans. Amer. Neurol. Ass.* 175 (1949).
12. FRENCH, J. D., VERZEANO, M. and MAGOUN, H. W., *Arch. Neurol. Psychiat.* **69**, 505 (1953).
13. LINDSLEY, D. F. and ADEY, W. R., *Exp. Neurol.* **4**, 358 (1961).
14. MORILLO, A. and BAYLOR, D., *Electroenceph. clin. Neurophysiol.* **15**, 455 (1963).
15. HIMWICH, H. E., MORILLO, A. and STEINER, W. G., *J. Neuropsychiat.* **3**, Suppl. 1, S15 (1962).
16. MORILLO, A., *Fed. Proc.* **21**, 346b (1962).
17. ADEY, W. R., DUNLOP, C. W. and SUNDERLAND, S., *J. comp. Neurol.* **110**, 173 (1958).
18. GELLHORN, E., *Physiological Foundations of Neurology and Psychiatry*, p. 351, University of Minnesota Press, Minneapolis (1953).
19. KLÜVER, H. and BUCY, P. C., *Arch. Neurol. Psychiat.* **42**, 979 (1939).
20. THOMSON, A. F. and WALKER, A. E., *Arch. Neurol. Psychiat.* **65**, 251 (1951).
21. FULLER, J. L., ROSVOLD, H. E. and PRIBRAM, K. H., *J. comp. physiol. Psychol.* **50**, 89 (1957).
22. SCHREINER, L. and KING, A., *J. Neurophysiol.* **16**, 643 (1953).
23. BRADY, J. B., Res. Rept. WRAIR-30-56, Walter Reed Army Medical Center, Washington D.C., 1956.
24. MACLEAN, P. D., *J. Nerv. ment. Dis.* **135**, 289 (1962).
25. HORNYKIEWICZ, O., In *Comparative Neurochemistry*, p. 379, Ed RICHTER, D., Pergamon Press, Oxford, 1964.
26. RINALDI, F. and HIMWICH, H. E., *Ann. N.Y. Acad. Sci.* **61**, 27 (1955).
27. RINALDI, F. and HIMWICH, H. E., *Dis. nerv. Syst.* **16**, 133 (1955).
28. STEINER, W. G., PSCHEIDT, G. R. and HIMWICH, H. E., *Science* **141**, 53 (1963).
29. PSCHEIDT, G. R., STEINER, W. G. and HIMWICH, H. E., *J. Pharmacol. exp. Ther.* **144**, 37 (1964).
30. RINALDI, F., RUDY, L. H. and HIMWICH, H. E., *Amer. J. Psychiat.* **112**, 678 (1956).
31. KILLAM, E. K. and KILLAM, K. F., In *Brain Mechanisms and Drug Action*, p. 71, Ed. FIELDS, W. J. Thomas, Springfield, 1957.
32. HIMWICH, H. E., In *Psychosomatic Medicine*, p. 211, Eds, NODINE, J. H. and MOYER, J. H., Lea and Febiger, Philadelphia, 1962.
33. BRADLEY, P. B. and ELKES, J., *Brain* **80** (1), 77 (1957).
34. STEINER, W. G. and HIMWICH, H. E., *Science* **136**, 873 (1962).
35. KOBAYASHI, T. and HIMWICH, H. E., *J. Neuropsychiat.* **5**, 123 (1963).
36. SARGANT, W., *J. Neuropsychiat.* **2**, S1, 1 (1961).

37. OVERALL, J. E., HOLLISTER, L. E., MEYER, F., KIMBELL, I. and SHELTON, J., *J. Amer. med. Ass.* In press.
38. COSTA, E., PSCHEIDT, G. R., VAN METER, W. G. and HIMWICH, H. E., *J. Pharmacol. exp. Ther.* **130**, 81 (1960).
39. DOYLE, C., STEINER, W. G. and HIMWICH, H. E., In preparation.
40. STEINER, W. G. and HIMWICH, H. E., *J. Nerv. ment. Dis.* **137**, 277 (1963).
41. HIMWICH, H. E., *Amer. Practit.* **11**, 687 (1960).
42. SCHALLEK, W. and KÜHN, A., *Proc. Soc. exp. Biol.* (*N.Y.*) **105**, 115 (1960).
43. MORILLO, A., REVZIN, A. M. and KNAUSS, T., *Psychopharmacologia* (*Berl.*) **3**, 386 (1962).
44. MORILLO, A., *Int. J. Neuropharmacol.* **1**, 353 (1962).
45. SCHWEIGERDT, E., SCHWEIGERDT, A. and HIMWICH, H. E., In preparation.
46. BONNYCASTLE, D. D., GIARMAN, N. J. and PAASONEN, M. K., *Brit. J. Pharmacol.* **12**, 228 (1957).
47. HUNT, H. F., *Ann. N.Y. Acad. Sci.* **67**, 712 (1957).
48. KLETZKIN, M. and BERGER, F. M., *Proc. Soc. exp. Biol.* (*N.Y.*) **100**, 681 (1959).
49. BONNYCASTLE, D. D., BONNYCASTLE, M. F. and ANDERSON, E. G., *J. Pharmacol. exp. Ther.* **135**, 17 (1962).
50. MASSERMAN, J. H., *Arch. Neurol. Psychiat.* **37**, 617 (1937).
51. KLEITMAN, N., *Sleep and Wakefulness.* University of Chicago Press, Chicago and London, 1963.

METHODS OF ASSESSMENT OF PSYCHOLOGICAL EFFECTS OF DRUGS IN ANIMALS*

HANNAH STEINBERG

Summary—The study of the effects of drugs on the behaviour of animals is interesting in its own right, but for the present purpose examples have been chosen which might be regarded as particularly relevant to psychiatry. Possible criteria of such relevance are discussed, and experiments on the following three topics are considered:

1. Experiments primarily concerned with time and dose relations, including experiments on potentiation, antagonism and toxicity.

2. Experiments concerned with selective effects of drugs on behaviour involving perception, learning and memory, as well as experiments concerned more directly with factors like " fear " and " stress ".

3. Experiments in which reasons for variability in reactions to drugs are analysed.

Résumé—L'étude des effets des médicaments sur le comportement des animaux est intéressante en elle même mais, ici, des examples qui peuvent paraître pertinents en psychiâtrie ont été choisis. Quelques critères d'un tel choix sont discutés et des expériences sur les trois sujets suivants sont considérées:

1. Expériences concernant les rapports entre effet, temps d'action et dosage y compris l'augmentation, l'antagonisme et la toxicité.

2. Expériences concernant l'effet sélectif des médicaments sur les aspects du comportement qui mettent en jeu la perception, l'apprentissage et la mémoire, ainsi que des expériences concernant plus particulièrement des facteurs tels que " la crainte " et " le stress ".

3. Expériences dans lesquelles les sources de variabilité dans les réactions aux médicaments sont analysées.

Zusammenfassung—Das Studium der Wirkung von Pharmaka auf das Verhalten von Tieren ist in sich selbst genügend interessant; im vorliegenden Falle jedoch wurden Beispiele gewählt, die als besonders bedeutsam für die Psychiatrie erscheinen. Es werden mögliche Kriterien einer solchen Bedeutsamkeit besprochen, und Versuche der folgenden drei Arten in Betracht gezogen:

1. Versuche, die in erster Linie Verhältnisse von Zeit und Dosis betreffen, einschliesslich Versuche, die Potenzierung, Antagonismus und Toxizität betreffen.

2. Versuche, die sich auf differenzielle Wirkungen von Pharmaka auf das Verhalten beziehen, das Wahrnehmung, Lernen und Gedächtnis einschliesst; sowie Versuche die direkt Faktoren wie " Furcht " und " Stress " betreffen.

3. Versuche, in denen Ursachen für die Variabilität der Reaktion auf die Pharmaka analysiert werden.

*The preparation of this paper was supported by research grant MH-03313 from the National Institute of Mental Health, U.S. Public Health Service.

THERE is a large and growing literature on the psychological effects of drugs in animals and on methods of assessing them. This work is intrinsically interesting, and it also yields basic information both about the mode of action of drugs and about the organization of behaviour. The first part of this review will briefly illustrate this. The second part will deal with animal experiments which might be regarded as specially relevant to psychiatry.

BASIC EXPERIMENTS

The following example is from the well-known work of Miller and his collaborators.[1, 2] Rats were trained in six different but related experimental set-ups to obtain a reward, either food or water, by running towards

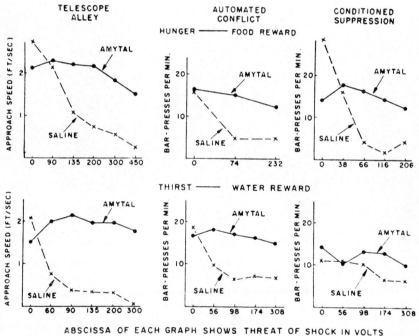

ABSCISSA OF EACH GRAPH SHOWS THREAT OF SHOCK IN VOLTS

FIG. 1. Effects of an intraperitoneal injection of 20 mg/kg of amylobarbitone sodium administered to Sprague–Dawley albino rats 20 min before testing in six experiments on fear and conflict using different techniques. The drug usually impaired performance while no electric shocks were given, but counteracted impairment when shocks occurred. (After Miller[1].)

it or by pressing levers. When they had learned this, the effects of amylobarbitone were studied, and it was found that animals given a fairly small dose of the drug usually ran more slowly or pressed a lever less often than control animals given saline (Fig. 1). Then the situations were changed so that the rats could only obtain the rewards if they also sometimes underwent punishment by means of electric shocks. As a result, the performance of un-drugged controls fell off markedly, but rats under the influence of the drug were little affected. Thus, under normal conditions amylobarbitone tended to impair performance, but in the presence of threats of punishment it improved it. A somewhat analogous reversal of the effects of barbiturates in man, incidentally, had been found by Hill, Belleville and Wikler[3]: a dose of pentobarbitone which normally increased reaction times actually decreased them when the subjects were given exceptionally high incentives to perform quickly. Miller's tentative explanation of the results shown in Fig. 1 was that amylobarbitone selectively mitigated the effects of punishment or " fear ", an interpretation which is not inconsistent with the clinical use of the drug. However, it was possible that the action was not directly on the behavioural mechanism concerned with fear, but was brought about in some other way, e.g. through impaired perception, discrimination or memory. These and other possibilities were tested and largely eliminated in a series of further analytical experiments. The " fear hypothesis " was also studied in another way. Rats were taught to inject themselves, by pressing a bar, with a solution of amylobarbitone, and it was found that their rate of self-injection increased markedly during periods when they were given electric shocks and presumably frightened

These animal experiments illustrate an important method of approach in psychopharmacology: to take a drug with known and useful clinical actions; to select tests of animal behaviour which attempt to mimic aspects of the clinical situation in which the drug is used; and to analyse whether the effects of the drug on the forms of behaviour so induced tally. In this way something can be learnt both about the mode of action of the drug, about the organization of punishment-induced behaviour and about the validity of the methods for studying it (cf. Steinberg[4]). The information so obtained may then also be used in the search for new drugs or new tests of behaviour.

However, what I should like to stress at this point is that even if the drug concerned had not been amylobarbitone, which is widely used clinically in the treatment of anxiety, and even if the behaviour had had nothing to do with punishments or fear which are at least superficially related to factors in human psychiatry, these experiments would still be of intrinsic and basic scientific interest. The same is true, I suggest, of many other kinds of animal experiments with drugs, for example, the analysis of sites of action of drugs in the brain by means of self-stimulation experiments,[5, 6] of the effects of drugs on learning and memory,[7] the interactions between drugs and eating and drinking,[8] the regulation of body temperature,[9] social behaviour[10] and so forth.

EXPERIMENTS SPECIALLY RELEVANT TO PSYCHIATRY

Much has been written about extrapolation from effects of drugs on animals to man,[11-15] and what follows is necessarily largely personal and reflects my own opinions and interests.

Some Criteria of Relevance

First a negative criterion. Superficial resemblance, or " face validity " as it is often called, is not automatically a reliable criterion. Many methods have been devised for animals which are modelled as directly as possible upon some, often rather global, conception of human mental illness. Most obvious examples are so-called " experimental neuroses " where incompatible stimuli or stimuli which are very difficult to discriminate are used to disrupt the behaviour of animals in various ways. This kind of experimental situation is probably much more complex than is sometimes realized,[16, 17] and the ability of a drug to mitigate such disturbed behaviour is not necessarily a reliable predictor of clinical efficacy in human neurosis. Benactyzine, for example, was reported particularly successful in such animal tests,[18] but seems to have been disappointing clinically.

Conversely, conditioned avoidance procedures, where animals are taught to make use of signals in order to avoid noxious stimuli, have shown themselves particularly sensitive to some phenothiazines and reserpine:[19] these drugs can abolish avoidance responses at doses which leave escape behaviour relatively unimpaired when the noxious stimuli actually do occur; and there is evidence which suggests that the potency of phenothiazines in this kind of experiment is correlated with their clinical potency.[20] Yet there is little obvious similarity between these experiments and the main use of phenothiazines which is to quieten acutely schizophrenic patients.

Although there are many promising correlations, it is probably true to say that there is as yet no single test of animal behaviour which can be regarded as a fairly certain predictor of a specific drug effect in psychiatric patients,[21] nor is it reasonable to expect this in the present state of our understanding of mental illness or the mode of action of drugs. A broader analytical step-by-step approach of the kind discussed under " Basic Experiments " seems to me therefore generally more appropriate. Another related criterion of relevance which I would recommend is the use of forms of animal behaviour about whose significance something is already understood, rather than procedures which are specially invented for the purpose of testing drugs; though one should of course observe the animal carefully before deciding which aspects of behaviour to select for further analysis. A corollary of this is that well studied animal species like rats, monkeys and mice are more likely to be useful than unusual animals like, for example, gerbils. Otherwise it is easier to put forward criteria of relevance by example than by general rule, and four topics are accordingly discussed below.

1. *Experiments Mainly Concerned with Dose and Time Relations*

The relative potencies and durations of action of different drugs can be compared by means of experiments on animal behaviour, and this is too well known to need illustration. Other effects which can be studied under this head are changes in the predominant effects of the same drug depending on the dose and on the time after administration. For example, barbiturates, like alcohol, are usually regarded, and rightly so, as general depressants of

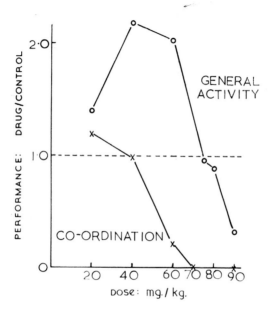

FIG. 2. Performance of mice given various doses of amylobarbitone sodium. Photocell activity cages were used to measure general activity, and a rotating rod on which the animals had to walk if they were not to fall off to measure co-ordination. (After Kinnard and Carr[22].)

most kinds of activity. Nevertheless it is well known clinically that sometimes, especially in small doses, effects which are more appropriately described as stimulant can be observed. Such stimulant effects can sometimes be demonstrated experimentally in man, and they have been shown conclusively in animals. For example, Kinnard and Carr[22] found increased general activity in mice with small doses of amylobarbitone but no improvement in a test of motor co-ordination at any dose (Fig. 2). Read, Cutting and Furst[23] found stimulant effects on general activity with some doses of phenobarbitone and alcohol early after injection but later effects became depressant. In both these cases there was a reversal of the direction of the effect in a particular test of behaviour which depended on the dose and/or the time since administration.

Potentiation and antagonism have long been important phenomena in general pharmacology,[24, 25] and the use of combinations of drugs in psychiatry is growing. Experiments on animal behaviour can sometimes provide a basis for their analysis. For example, my colleagues and I have recently studied the combined effects of various doses, in various ratios, of amphetamine and amylobarbitone.[26, 27] Mixtures of these two kinds of

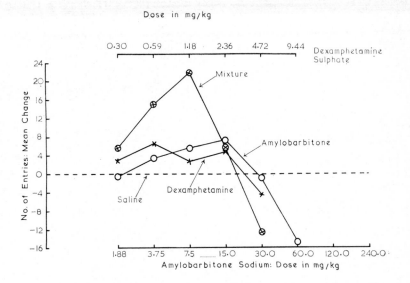

FIG. 3. Activity of rats influenced by dexamphetamine sulphate and amylobarbitone sodium, given separately and in combination, over a range of doses. The figure shows the number of entries into the arms of a Y-shaped runway during 5 min expressed as mean differences from the activity of the saline control group, the mean number of entries of which was 14·9, S.D. 7·4. Each point represents the mean results for a different group of eight rats. The ratio between the two drugs was kept constant at : 16·5, which is similar to " Drinamyl ". The peak mixture effect was greater than the sum of the effects of the ingredient doses and than the effect of any dose of the separate drugs.[27]

drugs have been used in psychiatry for many years, especially in the treatment of mild neuroses, but hardly any systematic work on their effects on the behaviour of animals—or of man—had, as far as we could discover, been done in the laboratory. Why such mixtures might be especially effective is not immediately obvious. Barbiturates in the fairly small doses used in psychiatry are usually intended to act as mild depressants or " sedatives ", though small doses of barbiturates can sometimes produce amphetamine-like effects in, for example, activity cages as has already been discussed. Amphetamine on the other hand is, of course, a cerebral stimulant, and its effects on most kinds of response tend to be the opposite of those of barbiturates.

Clinically, the effects of the two kinds of drug when given in combination have sometimes been described as " mutually corrective ",[28] that is, as somehow reinforcing each other's advantages while antagonizing each other's undesirable side actions. The manufacturers' literature particularly stresses favourable effects on the subjects' mood. The fact that the two drugs concerned are important drugs with well known and basic actions on the CNS was an additional reason for selecting mixtures of them for study.

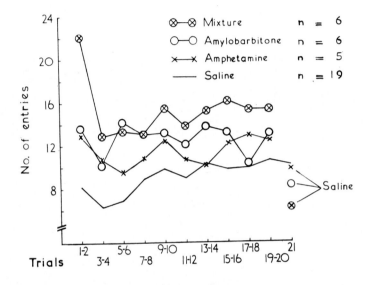

FIG. 4. Activity of four groups of rats tested under the influence of drugs at successive trials three days apart. The results have been grouped so that each point on the graph represents the mean of two successive trials. At the 21st trial all groups were tested with saline, and the high level of activity of the amphetamine-barbiturate mixture was not maintained.[33]

We used the amount of spontaneous " exploratory " activity by rats in a standard runway as one of the main measures. To our surprise, in some dose combinations the drugs had mutually potentiating effects: the increase in activity with these mixtures was much greater than the sum of the effects of the two ingredient doses, and also than the effect of *any* dose of the separate drugs. Figure 3 illustrates this potentiation for a dose ratio, by weight, of 1 : 6·5, which, incidentally, is the ratio used in the well-known " Drinamyl ". Further experiments showed that this marked potentiation occurred over a limited range of dose combinations which was distributed in an orderly fashion and could be plotted in the form of Loewe[29] diagrams or " isobols ". We also studied ataxia quantitatively, by determining the splay of the rats' footprints during a standard run.[30] Some mixtures which induced peak exploratory activity also produced marked ataxia, while others which produced equally high exploratory activity did not; and we found that whether or not ataxia occurred depended on the absolute amount of barbiturate in the mixture; mixtures containing less than 10 mg/kg amylobarbitone did not produce ataxia. The peak " Drinamyl " mixture shown in Fig. 3 was among those producing maximal exploratory activity with no ataxia—which is rather remarkable, since this ratio was, as far as we can discover, arrived at entirely on the basis of clinical observations.

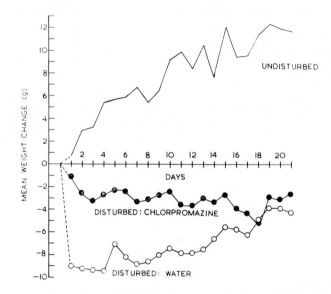

FIG. 5. Chlorpromazine inhibition of weight loss induced by removing rats to unfamiliar surroundings. Undisturbed rats remained in their usual surroundings throughout. The other two groups were moved to an unfamiliar environment at the beginning of the experiment; one group received 2 mg/kg chlorpromazine daily, the other a water control. Weight changes are expressed as mean gains or losses from the mean body weight of each group at the beginning of the experiment.[38]

A particularly interesting problem concerning time relations, which also leads into my second topic, is how far the behavioural effects induced by drugs persist after the drug has been withdrawn. This is of great importance clinically, where it is naturally desired to stop drugs as soon as possible. In most animal experiments, it has not been possible to demonstrate transfer from the drugged to the non-drugged state. For example, Bloch and Silva[31] found that what had been learned about a 4-unit T-maze while animals were under the influence of pentobarbitone was not retained when the animals were tested without the drug. Similarly Miller[2], in experiments on the experimental extinction of aversive behaviour induced by electric shocks, found that the beneficial effects of amylobarbitone did not remain when no drug was given. Hunt[32], had also failed to find transfer in somewhat similar experiments with chlorpromazine. We ourselves[33] found that the increased level of exploratory activity induced by an amphetamine-barbiturate mixture was not maintained when the drug was withdrawn (Fig. 4): activity without the drug was very low indeed. Ross and Schnitzer[34] on the other hand, found that rats which were under the influence of amphetamine sulphate during 45 min in activity cages were more active in these cages when retested without the drug a week later than control rats that had had their first exposure to the cages without any drug. Whether any transfer occurs or not must depend on quite complicated interactions between the drug and the conditions in which it is administered and withdrawn, and there is a great need for further analytical animal experiments. Otis[35] has recently suggested that if transfer is to occur the dose of drug administered must be large enough to modify existing habits while the drug is acting, but not so large as to block new learning during this time. Some of our own results[30] could be interpreted as consistent with this, since we have found that rats which had been given a drug mixture at their very first trial in a new environment seemed to behave at a second trial with saline as though their first trial had not occurred; but in rats which had had their first trial with saline, behaviour at the second trial was different.

2. " *Stress* ", " *Fear* " and " *Conflict* "

As one would expect, there is a large literature on the effects of drugs on the reactions of animals to noxious or conflicting stimuli, and there is not space to review it here. Experiments on " conditioned avoidance ", " experimental neurosis " and the methods used by Miller[1, 2] have already been referred to earlier. Many drugs can mitigate behavioural and physiological reactions to such stimuli in animals, as they can in man (cf. Steinberg[36]); though, as has already been suggested, it is often difficult to be sure that the effect is directly on fear or similar mechanisms, and is not brought about in some other way. It is perhaps worth noting that most animal experiments have made use of fairly violent stimuli, like electric shocks. Milder stimulation, e.g. changes of environment, can however, also elicit changes of behaviour, and these can also be modified by drugs.[26, 37, 38]

3. *Perception, Learning and Memory*

Perception. That changes of perception may be involved in psychiatric illnesses has long been recognized and has been demonstrated in experiments on thresholds, constancy and so forth. Similarly, it has been suggested that some drugs used in psychiatry may produce their beneficial effects primarily by altering perception in such a way that people are, for example, less easily disturbed by external stimuli. This kind of effect can be studied in animals. Weiskrantz[39], for example, has suggested that reserpine produces " behavioural non-reactivity " primarily by blocking sensory input, and he and his collaborators have tested this possibility in a series of experiments involving auditory perception and discrimination in monkeys; they concluded that it was the utilization of sensory information which seemed primarily affected by he drug.[40]

Learning and memory. One way of expressing the aims of psychiatric treatment is to say that it is intended to induce selective forgetting of undesirable old habits and the learning of desirable new ones. Therefore drugs which can improve or hinder learning and forgetting are at least potentially relevant. Jarvik[7] has recently reviewed the experimental evidence, mainly on animals, and has also considered effects in man.[41, 42] Reviews by Plotnikoff, Birzis, Mitoma, Otis, Weiss and Laties[43], and by Weiss and Laties[44], also contain many examples.

4. *Experiments on Individual Variability in Reaction to Drugs.*

Individual differences are one of the major problems in the psychiatric use of drugs. Attempts to study them systematically in a clinical setting can be very laborious and the results complicated and difficult to interpret.[45] In recent years there has been increasing interest in approaching them by laboratory experiments, both on man[46, 47] and on animals. Two main approaches can be distinguished:

(a) A correlational approach, in which the distribution of reactions in a group of unselected subjects is determined, and attempts are made to relate the individual differences which occur to other factors. For example Irwin, Slabok and Thomas[48] tested the spontaneous motor activity of rats with various doses of a number of drugs and concluded that an animal's sensitivity to drugs partly depended on its normal level of activity: naturally hyperactive rats tended to be relatively sensitive and hypoactive rats relatively insensitive to various drugs which increased or decreased motor activity. Similarly Kornetsky, Dawson and Pelikan[49] examined whether the degree of response of rats to various doses of one drug (pentobarbitone) was correlated with the degree of response of the same animals to various doses of another drug (dexamphetamine), using the rate of pressing levers for food rewards as a measure. They found very high correlations between response rates to different doses of the same drug, and somewhat lower though still very positive correlations between response rates with the two different drugs. This suggested that there might be something like " general drug sensitivity " in rats, and this is not inconsistent with results in experiments on man.[50]

(b) The second approach is to select or treat the experimental subjects beforehand in such a way as to maximize differences between groups of subjects. For example, it is now well known that amphetamine which is predominantly a cerebral stimulant can nevertheless be used to quieten over-excited children[51] but not adults. Attempts have been made to study this kind of effect in animals of different ages. Thus Heimstra and MacDonald[52] were not able to obtain anything suggesting sedation in young rats, possibly because they did not try to distinguish between " over excited " and " normal " young rats. They did, however, find some differences in behavioural re-actions according to age. In particular, older rats were made more " sociable " by amphetamine than younger rats as measured by the frequency of reactions to other rats. With some kinds of reaction, especially when rats differing very widely in age are studied, marked differential effects can

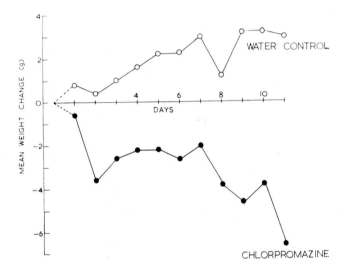

FIG. 6. Weight loss induced by chlorpromazine (2 mg/kg daily) in undisturbed rats—5 in each group (Watson and Steinberg, unpublished).

sometimes be determined. For example, Farner[53] has found that a dose of amphetamine which decreased food consumption of 27–30 months old rats by about 20 per cent, left that of rats aged up to 11 months unaffected.

Other factors which can markedly affect behavioural reactions to drugs in animals include species, strain, sex, temperature and, perhaps most relevant of all, the present and previous psychological circumstances of the animals. The increased toxicity of amphetamine when animals are crowded[54, 55] is now well known, and is probably due to a number of factors, including increased activity and higher body temperature.[56, 57] In man also the effects of drugs can be different according to whether they are administered in group or individual experiments.[58, 59] The previous experience of animals can sometimes make a decisive difference. For example, we[26] have found, in experiments with the amphetamine barbiturate mixtures already referred to, that a mixture which normally markedly stimulated exploratory activity completely failed to do this if the animals had had recent previous experience of the environment in which activity was being tested. We are at present trying to throw further light on this, for example, by studying the reactions to the drug mixtures in adult rats whose *infant* experiences had differed in various ways.

Other examples under this head are the reversal of the effects of amylobarbitone depending on whether rats were working under normal or frightening conditions already referred to[1, 2] and experiments on the effects of chlorpromazine on body weight, eating and drinking.[38] A small daily dose of chlorpromazine counteracted the loss of body weight in rats which had been disturbed by changes in their customary environment but in undisturbed rats the same drug treatment actually induced loss of body weight (Figs. 5 and 6). Such effects may link up with observations of weight changes when this drug is given clinically.[60] Animal experiments of this kind can sometimes be looked at in conjunction with experiments in man where reactions to drugs are systematically altered by expectation, instructions and so forth.[61]

CONCLUSION

There are many ways in which experiments on animal behaviour and drugs can be relevant to psychiatry, and only a few examples have been given in this review. Animal experiments make possible detailed and stepwise analyses of complex effects and the use of lengthy procedures and of wide ranges of doses and drugs. There is a great diversity of methods for assessing behavioural changes of drugs in animals, and how far results obtained by them with drugs are meaningful depends largely on the discrimination with which the methods are applied.[12, 62]

REFERENCES

1. MILLER, N. E., *Amer. Psychologist.* **16**, 12 (1961).
2. MILLER, N. E., In Steinberg, H., de Reuck, A. V. S. and Knight, J. ed. *Animal Behaviour and Drug Action*, p. 1. Churchill, London (1964).
3. HILL, H. E., BELLEVILLE, R. E. and WIKLER, A., *Arch. Neurol. Psychiat.* **77**, 28 (1957).
4. STEINBERG, H., *Acta Psychologica.* **19**, 771 (1961).
5. OLDS, J., In Ramey, E. R. and O'Doherty, D. S. ed. *Electrical Studies on the Unanesthetized Brain*, p. 17. Hoeber–Harper, New York (1960).
6. STEIN, L., In Steinberg, H., de Reuck, A. V. S. and Knight, J. ed. *Animal Behaviour and Drug Action*, p. 91. Churchill, London (1964).
7. JARVIK, M., In Steinberg, H., de Reuck, A. V. S. and Knihgt, J. ed. *Animal Behaviour and Drug Action*, p. 44. Churchill, London (1964)
8. ANDERSSON, B. and LARSSON, S., *Pharmacol. Rev.* **13**, 1 (1961).
9. WEISS, B. and LATIES, V. G., *J. Pharmacol.* **140**, 1 (1963).
10. CHANCE, M. R. A. and SILVERMAN, A. P., In Steinberg H., de Reuck, A. V. S. and Knight, J. ed. *Animal Behaviour and Drug Action*, p. 65. Churchill, London (1964),

11. Evarts, E. V., In Cole, J. O. and Gerard, R. W. ed. *Psychopharmacology: Problems in Evaluation*, p. 284. National Academy of Sciences—National Research Council, Washington (1958).
12. U.S. Department of Health, Education and Welfare, Public Health Service. Behavioral Research in Preclinical Psychopharmacology. No. 968 (1962).
13. Irwin, S., In Steinberg, H., de Reuck, A. V. S. and Knight, J. ed. *Animal Behaviour and Drug Action*, p. 280. Churchill, London (1964).
14. Steinberg, H., de Reuck, A. V. S. and Knight, J. ed., *Animal Behaviour and Drug Action*. Churchill, London (1964).
15. Russell, R. W., *Ann. Rev. Psychol.* 15, 87 (1964).
16. Russell, R. W., *Brit. J. Psychol.* 41, 95 (1950).
17. Waters, R. H., Rethlingshafer, D. A. and Caldwell, W. E. ed., *Principles of Comparative Psychology*. McGraw-Hill, New York (1960).
18. Jacobsen, E. and Skaarup, Y., *Acta Pharm. Tox., Kbh.* 11, 125 (1955).
19. Dews, P. B. and Morse, W. H., *Ann. Rev. Pharmacol.* 1, 145 (1961).
20. Cook, L. and Kelleher, R. T., *Ann. Rev. Pharmacol.* 3, 205 (1963).
21. Riley, H. and Spinks, A., *J. Pharm., Lond.* 10, 657 and 721 (1958).
22. Kinnard, W. J. and Carr, C. J., *J. Pharmacol.* 121, 354 (1957).
23. Read, G., Cutting, W. and Furst, A., *Psychopharmacologia* 1, 346 (1960).
24. Veldstra, H., *Pharmacol. Rev.* 8, 339 (1956).
25. Gaddum, J. H., In Rothlin, E. ed., *Neuropsychopharmacology* 2, p. 19. Elsevier, Amsterdam (1960).
26. Steinberg, H., Rushton, R. and Tinson, C., *Nature (Lond.).* 192, 533 (1961).
27. Rushton, R. and Steinberg, H., *Brit. J. Pharmacol.* 21, 295 (1963).
28. Myerson, A., *New Eng. J. Med.* 221, 561 (1939).
29. Loewe, S., *Ergebn. Physiol.* 27, 47 (1928).
30. Rushton, R., Steinberg, H. and Tinson, C., *Brit. J. Pharmacol.* 20, 99 (1963).
31. Bloch, S. and Silva, A., *J. comp. Physiol. Psychol.* 52, 550 (1959).
32. Hunt, H. F., In *Conference on Drugs and Psychiatry*, National Research Council, Washington, D.C. (1956).
33. Rushton, R. and Steinberg, H., In Steinberg, H., de Reuck, A. V. S. and Knight, J. ed., *Animal Behaviour and Drug Action*, p. 207. Churchill, London (1964).
34. Ross, S. and Schnitzer, S. B., *Psychol. Rep.* 13, 461 (1963).
35. Otis, L., *Proc. IV International Congress of Neuropsychopharmacology* (1964). (In the press)
36. Steinberg, H., *Brit. med. Bull.* 20, 75 (1964).
37. Broadhurst, P. L., Sinha, S. N. and Singh, S. D., *J. genetic. Psychol.* 95, 217 (1959).
38. Steinberg, H. and Watson, R. H. J., *Proc. physiol. Soc.* 147, 20 (1959).
39. Weiskrantz, L., In Garattini, S. and Ghetti, V. ed., *Psychotropic Drugs*, p. 67. Elsevier, Amsterdam (1957).
40. Gross, C. G. and Weiskrantz, L., *Quart. J. exp. Psychol.* 13, 34 (1961).
41. Summerfield, A. and Steinberg, H., *Quart. J. exp. Psychol.* 9, 146 (1957).
42. Summerfield, A. and Steinberg, H., In Bradley, P. B., Denniker, P. and Radouco-Thomas, C. ed., *Neuropsychopharmacology*, p. 481. Elsevier, Amsterdam (1959).
43. Plotnikoff, N., Birzis, L., Mitoma, C., Otis, L., Weiss, B. and Laties, V., Psychological Sciences Division, Office of Naval Research, Washington (1960).
44. Weiss, B. and Laties, V. G., *Pharmacol. Rev.* 14, 1 (1962).
45. Hamilton, M., Hordern, A., Waldrop, F. N. and Lofft, J., *Brit. J. Psychiat.* 109, 510 (1963).
46. Lindemann, E. and Felsinger, J. M., *Psychopharmacologia* 2, 69 (1961).
47. Eysenck, H. J., *Experiments with Drugs*. Pergamon Press, London (1963).
48. Irwin, S., Slabok, M. and Thomas, G., *J. Pharmacol.* 123, 206 (1958).
49. Kornetsky, C., Dawson, J. and Pelikan, E., In Rinkel, M. ed., *Specific and Non-Specific Factors in Psychopharmacology*, p. 161. Philosophical Library, New York (1963).
50. Kornetsky, C., In Uhr, L. and Miller, J. G. ed., *Drugs and Behavior*, p. 297. Wiley, New York (1960).

51. BRADLEY, C., *Pediatrics, Springfield.* **5**, 24 (1950).
52. HEIMSTRA, N. W. and MCDONALD, A., *Psychopharmacologia* **3**, 212 (1962).
53. FARNER, VON D., *Gerontologia* **5**, 35 (1961).
54. GUNN, J. A. and GURD, M. R., *J. Physiol.* **97**, 453 (1940).
55. CHANCE, M. R. A., *J. Pharmacol.* **87**, 214 (1946).
56. HOEHN, R. and LASAGNA, L., *Psychopharmacologia, Berl.* **1**, 210 (1960).
57. HARDINGE, M. G. and PETERSON, D. I., *J. Pharmacol.* **145**, 47 (1964).
58. NOWLIS, V. and NOWLIS, H. H., *Ann. N.Y. Acad. Sci.* **65**, 345 (1956).
59. JOYCE, C. R. B., *Proc. Soc. Psychosomatic Research.* Pergamon Press, London. (In the press.)
60. CRISP, A. H., *Proc. VI International Congress of Psychotherapy, London.* (In the press.)
61. PENNICK, S. and FISHER, S., *Report for Psychopharmacology Service Center, National Institute of Mental Health.* (In the press.)
62. DEWS, P. B., In Bachrach, A. J. ed., *Experimental Foundations of Clinical Psychology.* Basic Books (1962).

METHODS OF ASSESSMENT OF PSYCHOLOGICAL EFFECTS OF DRUGS IN MAN

MAX HAMILTON

Summary—(1) The selection of patients determines the accuracy versus the generality of inferences. (2) The method of assessment determines the accuracy versus the difficulty of measurement. (3) The aim of the investigation determines the type of data used and the method of analysis.

Rèsumè—(1) La sélection des patients détermine la précision des résultats. (2) La méthode d'évaluation est un autre facteur qui contribue à la précision des résultats. (3) Le but de l'expérimentation détermine le choix des critères et la méthode d'analyse.

Zusammenfassung—(1) Von der Auswahl der Patienten hängt es ab, wie zutreffend die Schlussfolgerungen sind, die aus einer klinischen Untersuchung gezogen werden können. (2) Geeignete Auswertungsmethoden ermöglichen eine richtige Beurteilung trotz schwerer Messbarkeit der Ergebnisse. (3) Das Ziel der Untersuchung bestimmt die Art der auszuwertenden Daten und die analytische Methode.

INTRODUCTION

The psychological effects of drugs in man can be considered from the narrow therapeutic point of view, in which the main interest is their effects in the treatment of mental disorder and from the more general viewpoint of the psychopharmacologist, who is interested in the effects of drugs on higher activity of the central nervous system. It is the former which will be considered here, although only slight modifications of the statements to be made would be needed to cover the more general aspects of the problem.

After the usual pharmacological investigation of the effect of a drug on animals, the assessment in man must pass through two stages. The first of which consists of a preliminary try-out on human subjects and patients, preferably based on indications arising from the experiments on animals but designed to present as wide a range of phenomena or symptoms as possible to elicit effects of the drug to be observed. On this basis, hypotheses about the nature of the psychological effects can be made and these should be tested by the second stage: the controlled trial.

The assessment of drugs without the controlled trial has now been made old-fashioned by the advance of scientific method and bitter experience has shown that such inadequate methods must now be regarded as uninformative, misleading and even dangerous. They are uninformative because without the base-line provided by the control group, results cannot be compared with

39

those of other treatments. They are misleading because, as is now well known, the results obtained reflect the enthusiasm of the investigators more than the effects of the drugs. They are dangerous because, by encouraging the use of ineffective drugs, they inhibit the development and application of better ones.

Many accounts have been published giving the underlying basis of clinical trials and the practical problems involved.[1, 2] It will be assumed here that such fundamentals are understood and accepted and therefore this paper will be concerned with some detailed aspects of three problems in the organization of a controlled trial.

SELECTION OF PATIENTS

A controlled trial is essentially a comparison of the effects of two or more drugs on an appropriate number of comparable groups of patients and, given a positive result, it will be concluded that one of the treatments was better than the other, or others, in those groups. These results will be used to infer that similar results will be obtained on further *groups* of patients, *selected in the same way*. It is obvious enough that the patients subsequenˈly to be given the drug must be selected in the same way as those in the original trial but it is insufficiently realized that inferences on the value of the drug apply only to *groups* of patients. The physician engaged in clinical practice, however, is concerned with individual patients not with groups. Hence, the value of such inferences in the treatment of patients depends inversely on the variability (or heterogeneity) of the group.

The more accurate the definition of the group, the less will be its variability and the more useful will be the inferences. " Definition " means here the adequate categorization of the factors which determine the response to treatment. For example, if the sex of the patient is an important factor in determining the outcome of treatment then, if the original group contained both sexes, i.e. the group did not consist of patients of a defined sex, then it will be less easy to predict the outcome for a patient of particular sex. The same applies to such other factors as age, diagnosis, constitution, length of history of illness, etc., provided these are factors determining the outcome. If the group has been adequately defined in terms of such factors, then it will be possible to select patients (or subjects) in the future and to predict accurately their reponse to treatment but no inference can be made about patients who do not come within the bounds of the definitions. Thus, accurate delimitation of the type of patient improves the prediction from the results of the trial but limits its range of application.

In planning a trial, therefore, the investigator has to strike a balance between these two limits. Practical considerations also play a part here. If the patients come from a wide range of types, then it is easy to accumulate sufficient numbers for the trial which can then be completed in a reasonable time whereas, if the patients are selected within narrowly defined limits, the accumulation of cases will proceed slowly and the trial will be excessively prolonged. The investigator will have to decide whether he wants some sort of answer to his question quickly or whether he would prefer to wait longer to get a better answer. In this connection, it must be remembered that a heterogeneous group has great variability. This (technically, the variance) acts as the denominator when assessing the statistical significance of the difference between the groups so a great variability will more readily yield a null result. In clinical terms, this means that a particular subgroup of patients may be the one that responds to the treatment, and this may be lost, by dilution, in the total group. A narrowly defined group will have a smaller variance, and will thus be capable of being more sensitive to the statistical test, but the narrow definition may also exclude the specifically " sensitive " group.

These difficulties may be solved by replicating the investigation on all the narrowly defined groups, but clearly, this entails using much larger numbers of patients and may indefinitely prolong the experiment. Human nature being what it is, it is very disheartening to be involved in much work for a long time and yet see no results.

ASSESSMENT OF PSYCHOLOGICAL CHANGES

The measurement of psychological changes can be classified into four types:

(a) Overall improvement.

(b) Check lists and questionnaires.

(c) Ratings of symptoms and behaviour.

(d) Physiological changes accompanying clinical changes.

The first three can be done by the patients themselves or by others; the two ways will serve to check on each other.

Judging overall improvement is comparatively simple and easy but suffers from the fact that it is a very coarse method. Large numbers of patients may have to be used in order to improve the accuracy of the mean change for the purpose required. The use of check lists and questionnaires is much more accurate and sensitive. In the first place, they give information on the qualitative aspects of improvement (and worsening) in that particular items of behaviour and symptoms are recorded. The results can also be summed in some appropriate way to give an overall index of change. A number of difficulties may arise when patients use these devices for self-assessment. The patients may be too ill to fill in the forms properly. They may misunderstand them owing to regional and class differences in the use of words and, for various reasons, they may give incorrect answers, either to mislead themselves or their physicians. For example, a patient may be reluctant to admit how ill he is, or that he has certain symptoms or he may be anxious to convince others that he really is ill, and exaggerate his symptoms.

The rating of symptoms and behaviour is one of the best methods but is difficult to achieve satisfactorily because it needs well-trained raters. It also requires good rating scales and there is considerable room for improvement here. Rating scales for symptoms of schizophrenia are far from satisfactory and the rating of behaviour in this disorder is too sensitive to cultural and environmental factors. Finally, the measurement of physiological changes has the advantage of giving unbiased instrumental recordings but these must be proved to be valid, i.e. that they measure changes that are relevant in the given context of the investigation. Furthermore, it must be shown that the drugs used do not interfere with such measurements by reason of their effects on the peripheral nervous system. For example, it is known that some depressives have greatly diminished salivary secretion compared with normal subjects. A drug might improve the patient's clinical state but, by reason of an atropine-like effect, prevent the salivary secretion from increasing parallel with the improvement. Alternatively, a pilocarpine-like effect might increase salivary secretion without affecting the clinical state.

MEASURE OF IMPROVEMENT

At the end of the investigation, there will be available, for two or more treatments, some sort of score for each patient, both before and after the treatment. There may be a set of scores for each patient, but only the univariate case will be considered here. How is this data to be examined in order to come to a conclusion on the effects of the drugs?

The statistical test will determine the significance of the difference in scores after the various treatments, and this will depend inversely on the variability (variance) of the scores. Some of this variance may arise from the variance of the initial scores. To take an extreme hypothetical case, the treatment may have resulted in a drop of about 4, say, points for all patients. The variance of " after " scores would therefore be much the same as the " before " scores, and most of it would be eliminated by using " difference " scores, i.e. by subtracting " after " scores from " before " scores, and using these for the statistical test. It is important to understand the implications of the use of " difference " scores. In the first place, it assumes that the drug has the same effect regardless of the initial state of the patients. This may not be true, for the effect of the drug may depend on the initial score, i.e. severely ill patients may respond better than mildly ill patients, or vice versa. Secondly, the use of " difference " scores assumes that changes at different levels are equivalent. For example, it assumes that a change from 30 to 25 points is equivalent to a change from 5 to 0 points.

Instead of using " difference " scores, the data could be analysed by doing an analysis of co-variance on the final scores. This statistical technique has the effect of " adjusting " the final scores to the level they would have had, had all the initial scores been equal (at the average score). This method assumes that the relationship between initial and final scores is the same for all treatments. This may be quite untenable in some circumstances, e.g. when a drug is being tested against a placebo. It is true that one begins with the null hypothesis, that the drug has no more effect than the placebo, which implies that the relation between initial and final scores is the same for both treatments, but the net effect is that there are now two null hypotheses where the investigator intended to examine only one. There are other difficulties, but these are rarely important in clinical practice. Analysis of co-variance should not be done on " difference " scores, because of spurious correlations.[3]

Another scoring method is to use for the statistical test, the ratio between initial and final scores. Such ratio scores have the advantage that they equate patients who make the same proportional recoveries, and this is particularly appropriate in some circumstances for they equate complete recoveries, regardless of the initial state of the patient, severely or mildly ill. This is in accord with clinical practice. The disadvantage of ratio scores is that they equate patients with different final scores. Thus 30/60 is a 50 per cent recovery and is treated as equivalent to 5/10, but this ignores the fact that the first patient after treatment is very ill in comparison with the first before treatment.* It may be added that the distribution of ratio scores may be such that ordinary statistical tests may become inappropriate.

All these difficulties may be resolved by dividing the patients into groups according to the level of score before treatment, e.g. high, medium and low, and then doing a two-way analysis of variance on the final scores. Not only does this technique provide evidence about the relation between initial and final scores but it also shows whether this differs between the drugs and does this without any underlying assumptions. The only difficulty is that the experiment becomes much more complicated and introduces all the practical problems mentioned above.

In effect, there are a number of ways in which the improvement in patients may be measured and the data analysed. Each one involves certain assumptions which must be accepted or rejected according to the aims of the investigation.

REFERENCES

1. HAMILTON, M., *Lectures on the Methodology of Clinical Research*, Livingstone, Edinburgh, 1961.
2. SAINSBURY, P. and KREITMAN, N. B., *Methods of Psychiatric Research*, Oxford University Press, London, 1963.
3. OLDHAM, P. D., *J. chron. Dis.* **15**, 969 (1962).

* The figures have been selected to demonstrate the point whether the ratio is Before/After or After/Before.

DISCUSSION

OPENER: A. SUMMERFIELD:

I am sure you will agree that we have heard three papers which were not only of exceptional individual interest but covered a very considerable part of the spectrum of the problem. It is not, therefore, altogether a straightforward matter for a discussant to interrelate the three. I propose to refer briefly to the papers themselves, but to add some ideas of my own which may serve to interrelate the kinds of problems which are the subject of the three papers.

The interest in drugs of all those present is concerned with relationships between behaviour and the central nervous system, where these drugs exert some of their principal effects. It was, therefore, of the greatest interest to hear from Dr. Himwich, of the sort of progress which is being made in knowledge about where in the central nervous system drugs act. The controversial point that I want to make is that while this is necessary, it is by no means sufficient. Since we are concerned with the correlation between behaviour and drug action it is essential and necessary that our understanding of behaviour itself should be advanced. Progress on both fronts is essential for the development of the correlation.

The second point that I want to make is that when we are concerned with effects of drugs on behaviour, there are several components which are all interacting. An understanding of each, therefore, becomes necessary.

I should, therefore, like to advance a simple scheme of what it seems to me is the situation when drugs are used in psychiatry. Having put this forward, I want to show how this scheme can be used to represent the situation in drug experiments whether on animals or on humans.

In psychiatry we must consider the patient: the patient has a variety of characteristics about which one should know. There is, for example, the sex, the age, the past history of the patient. Secondly, if we use drugs to treat patients we must consider characteristics of these drugs, for example, the dose, the length of time they act, and the frequency of administration.

However, the administration of a certain drug in a certain fashion is one of the sets of variable conditions acting on the patient. There are all the other therapeutic procedures which are involved in the care of the patient whether it is individual treatment, institutional care and so on. Thus there are at least two sets of influences on any patient. The object is to produce a desirable change in the behaviour of the patient.

Similar interactions of such conditions are involved in experimental studies. There is the subject of the experiment whether animal or human, and the subject will have its own characteristics. In some experiments, particularly those in animals, it is possible to control some of those characteristics to a reasonable extent, e.g. its past history. In experiments on man this is exceedingly difficult to do except in a limited sense.

Ideally we are seeking to study effects of doses of drugs in the experiments. We must however, recognize three other influences which effect experiments on man.

(1) First of all we must tell the subject what we are doing. We must give him a task (psychological test, intelligence test, lever pressing, etc.) and we must give him instructions of some kind in relation to the task.

(2) We must consider the duration of changes that might be involved. In one type of experiment we are concerned only with the change in the subject's performance of the same task with and without the drug. The second type of investigation is that which involves learning on the part of the subject. In this case a continued change in the behaviour of the subject after the experimental procedure is one of the things which is of interest. This second type of experiment is in many ways more analogous to the multiple conditions scheme, since in learning experiments one is in some way interfering with the history, but not the future of the subject of the experiment. Thus experiments involving learning are, perhaps, more relevant to the therapeutic situation.

There is no doubt that experiments on the human involving learning, except in limited situations, are very much more difficult than experiments which involve a simple study of changed responses to tasks which may be attributed to the drugs.

In order to make progress in this field it is necessary to be concerned with the actual behaviour. I want to consider this by reference to some very simple forms of behaviour to the performance rather than of learning type. Most studies of the effects of drugs have involved simple tasks to assess performance. For example, are the movements of a person slowed down by a given drug? Here the normal behaviour has simply been the rate at which the subject has been able to tap the morse key. Other measurements attempt to answer the question, " Are movements less accurate? " These require the study of accuracy of aiming a stylus at a moving target. A third measures reaction time to determine whether reactions are slower. Alternatively, impairment of mental processes can be studied with tasks like the speed and accuracy with which the subject can do arithmetic.

While these tasks seem simple, from a psychological point of view they are not. If we consider the " simple " task involving rates of tapping a morse key. In some experiments undertaken by Dr. Steinberg the subject was instructed to tap a morse key as fast as he could. A comparison was made between doing this task with no drug and after having been given 15 mg of amphetamine sulphate. With amphetamine sulphate the subject will produce an appreciably higher rate of tapping than those obtained in control observations without the drug. This change is maintained over time so that it is possible to get curves of the time course of action of the drug in terms of this measure. Then a seemingly slight difference in the terms of the experiment was made—on the instructional input. At the end of each test the subject was given his score. Thus the next time he did the task he had information about how well he did the previous time. When this was done no difference could be found between amphetamine and the control. Giving the subject information about his performance is, perhaps motivating and providing incentive and even without the drug the subject goes on getting better. If the drug is given as well this has no further additional effect. Thus even in apparently simple sorts of performance tests details of conditions can make radical differences to the results. These will in turn make radical differences to inference about the effects of the drug.

In order to gain more information there are two methods of generalizing in connection with drug experiments. The first is to look to the tasks and to seek to analyse them from a psychological point of view. The second one studies different drugs and makes comparisons between their effects on the same kind of performance. Thus, for example, if we examine chlorpromazine and barbiturates, using similar tasks we shall find disjunctive effects. That is to say cases where chlorpromazine produces an impairment of one task where a barbiturate does not but with a second related task at the same dose and conditions the effects are reversed. This provides the opportunity of seeking to understand the actions of the drugs on behaviour in terms of the psychological difference between the tasks that are involved.

Experiments on effects of drugs on behaviour must, therefore, be undertaken with great care in the determination of the psychological conditions, both in the subject and imposed by the test for valid conclusions to be drawn.

OPENER: IAN OSWALD:

When I was invited to act as an opener of the discussion on the basic concepts involved in drug study in psychiatry, it was stressed that I was at liberty to extend my remarks outside the field of the main speakers.

The speakers have concerned themselves primarily with the direct effects of drugs during the period of their administration. I feel that it is important to realize that when we give a drug and then stop it, the effects of its administration do not cease at the time when the drug has been eliminated from the tissues. It is this basic concept that I want to discuss. In her paper Dr. Steinberg showed two figures, one from Miller, and one of her own in which the rats given amphetamine-barbiturate mixtures or barbiturates alone were stimulated. Examination of that data shows that when the drugs were stopped, the activity of the animals returned not to the base-line but below it for a period. It is this aspect that I want to discuss. By giving the drug for a period of time we may have induced unnatural changes in the patterns of central nervous system metabolism that can need weeks for their reversal.

We are by now all familiar with long time-lags in relation to drugs used in psychiatry. Give a patient a barbiturate by mouth and it takes effect in 30 min. Give imipramine and there may be a time-lag of 2 weeks before benefit. We are learning that, having given a monoamine oxidase inhibitor, the patient may be abnormally sensitive to certain other drugs for two or three weeks after stopping the monoamine oxidase inhibitor. By contrast with these drugs, the sleeping pills are thought of as drugs with an evanescent action, here tonight and gone tomorrow.

Yet we see so many patients, whom we would not call barbiturate addicts, who just take a couple of sleeping pills each night, and who are extremely resistant to any suggestion that they should give them up. We learn from them that these pills were started, often in hospital, 5 or 10 years ago and have never been stopped. " I've tried to stop them, doctor, but I just can't sleep properly without them." And so it goes on year after year, and 10 per cent of all N.H.S. general practitioner prescriptions are for sleeping pills. Five hundred million sleeping pills a year in England and Wales—excluding hospital and private prescribing. One wonders how many prescriptions are given at private consultations because the regular N.H.S. practitioner refuses to accede to further requests for the beloved sleeping pills.

Is it solely a psychological dependence, has the patient merely learned that swallowing the pills opens a quick avenue to oblivion? Or has her physiology been changed, so that the drug is now woven inextricably into her brain chemistry so that, if the drug were suddenly lacking, a violent biochemical perturbation would arise?

A couple of years ago Dr. Thacore and I were studying the sleep of women addicted to amphetamine and a dexamphetamine-amylobarbitone mixture. They had taken these drugs for so long that their nervous systems seemed to have adjusted to the presence of these drugs to the extent of allowing practically normal sleep. But when we suddenly stopped their drugs their sleep became suddenly very abnormal, and return to normal function took up to two months (Fig. 1).[1]

What of people of normal personality, put on to moderate doses of sleeping pills? Does their metabolism adjust to the pills so that the drugs lose their initial effect, at the same time creating a physiological dependence on the drugs? Dr. R. Priest and I have been doing an experiment using a new non-barbiturate sleeping pill, Ro 4-5360 (1,3-dihydro-7-nitro-5-phenyl-

2H-1,4-benzodiazepin-2-one).* I am confident from previous, less elaborate, research that our results would not have differed had we used a barbiturate.

We used two senior undergraduate volunteers during their long vacation. Covering about 12 miles of paper we recorded their EEGs throughout nineteen nights. First we did five base-line night recordings. Then the sleeping drug was given nightly for two weeks. They both reported very sound, pleasant, dreamless sleep, but with hangovers (on the fairly heavy dose of 15 mg). As the nights went by, they adjusted to the foreign chemicals, and

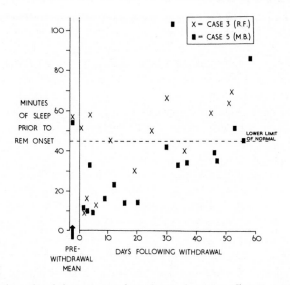

FIG. 1. Rebound and slow recovery from dexamphetamine (Case 3) and Drinamyl (Case 5). Depicted are delays between first falling asleep and first onset of paradoxical or rapid eye movement (REM) sleep, normally never less than 45 min.
    After drug withdrawal grossly abnormal values occur and not until after the 47th day did Case 5 show consecutive values within normal limits.

noticed a decrease of hangover and return of dreaming. Then we stopped their pills. They then noticed, for a few days, a slight shakiness with restlessness and dreaming (including a nightmare) at night.

Among the other sleep functions we were able to measure easily was the proportion of each night spent in the " paradoxical phase " of sleep. We now know that sleep is of two kinds, quite distinct in physiological characteristics which alternate during the night and of each of which a fairly fixed ration is normally needed to maintain normal brain function.[2]

On the base-line nights they averaged 24·3 per cent of paradoxical sleep, a very normal figure. On starting the drug, this fell at once to 7 per cent which

---

* Details of the study will be published elsewhere when complete.

is so low as to be quite abnormal, but as the nights went by the proportion climbed gradually up again towards the base-line mean. Then, after 2 weeks we stopped the drugs and a tremendous " rebound ", maximal on the third night after stopping the drug occurred when they averaged 35 per cent (a value so high as to be quite abnormal). Gradually over the next 2 weeks, the proportion of paradoxical sleep fell down, gently towards the base-line once more. Two weeks on the drugs. Two weeks to recover from the drugs. Giving them those sleeping pills did something to their brains from which they took a long time to recover.

No doubt there are hundreds of other physiological functions which we cannot measure which would give a similar picture of adjustment and rebound-with-slow-recovery. If this is so, one can begin to realize the violent repercussions that sudden stopping of a simple sleeping pill can have on a nervous system adjusted thereto, and why people are so loath to renounce their pills.

I believe we should caution both ourselves and our colleagues in other specialities before starting a patient on sleeping pills. When the time comes to stop, physiological recovery may take weeks. Psychological recovery may sometimes never occur, for the patient has learned a quick-escape habit.

REFERENCES

1. OSWALD, I. and THACORE, V. R., *Brit. med. J.* **ii**, 427 (1963).
2. OSWALD, I., In *Scientific Basis of Medicine. Annual Reviews 1964*, p. 102, Athlone Press, London.

GENERAL DISCUSSION

H. E. Himwich: I enjoyed the invited discussants' remarks very much and I agree with Dr. Summerfield that the studies such as I made are only some of many facets. I would also agree with Dr. Oswald's worry about the amount of psychoactive drugs administered. This is true for the United States, too. Outside hospitals, about one-third of all prescriptions for psychoactive drugs are for chlordiazepoxide, a slightly smaller fraction for meprobamate. The phenothiazines are also about 30 per cent of which chlorpromazine accounts for about half. The other drugs used made up the remaining 10 per cent.

He was absolutely right in saying that it was obvious from his work that drugs changed people and changed them fundamentally. I would also like to offer the thought that perhaps these people have warped metabolism initially, in fact many people are now working on the possible theory that people are schizophrenics because of a defect in their metabolism. So you are not starting necessarily on a normal metabolism and a drug may be working on a metabolism which is already disturbed.

J. R. Smythies: I wish to make two comments on what Dr. Oswald was saying and to ask Dr. Steinberg a question. In respect of the long-term effect of drugs Dr. Oswald mentioned the effect of the sleeping pills and amphetamine. In rats Takahashi and Akabane[1] in Japan showed that methamphetamine given daily for 25–57 days caused a depression in the level of activity of brain hexokinase. After this they took a month to return to normal levels. Administration for less than 25 days did not produce this effect. Interestingly they report that brain hexokinase activity was similarly depressed in brain biopsy specimens from schizophrenics.

The other drug which appears to have long-term effects is mescaline. I have seen several clinical cases in which one dose of mescaline has produced effects 2–3 weeks later under certain circumstances. In one particular case, a normal person, very little reaction occurred at the time. Three weeks later he went to Spain, and slept very little; he arrived exhausted on the airport and suddenly experienced a full blown mescaline reaction lasting about 6 hr.

I would like to ask Dr. Steinberg about one particular animal test which has been widely used; namely, the test of rats climbing ropes—you teach the rat that there is food at the top of the rope and measure the time that it takes to climb it. Does she think that some of the results can be explained on the basis not of behaviour differences but on muscle activity depression? The amount of muscular work involved is obviously great.

Russell Barton (*Colchester*): I should like to criticize one aspect of Dr. Steinberg's paper which is I believe fundamental in a symposium entitled " scientific aspects ". She has expressed the results of animal experiments in terms of subjective experience—i.e. she has assumed that rats feel fear. I would suggest that we have only circumstantial evidence for this. All her results could be explained equally easily on other grounds, e.g. that the drug caused nausea and that preoccupation with this caused behaviour differences.

I think it is most important that we distinguish between scientific basis and conjecture. That we express the results clearly and avoid assumptions based on our own subjective experience.

D. C. Watt (*Aylesbury*): I would like to take up the fourth of Professor Hamilton's methods of determining drug effects. He called this " physiological measures " but I believe it can be more appropriately called " physiological correlates ". Measure suggests accurate estimations based on knowledge of aetiology, e.g. blood sugar in diabetes. Such physiological determinations would be very valuable in psychiatry and might enable us to dispense with the less accurate clinical assessment. Nevertheless, they are not based on knowledge of pathology of the disorder and the term " measure " is therefore misleading.

J. M. HINTON (*London*): May I disagree with Dr. Watt. I fully agree with calling it a physiological " measure ". This is done because if you keep the term physiological measure you know that you are measuring something—may be pulse, blood pressure, or whatever it may be and it is confined to that measure. A " correlate " makes an assumption that there is a correlation between the physiological effect and the psychological state of that person. I think that throughout these experiments one should confine oneself to the measure and on the basis of further information decide if it is a correlate or not.

D. C. WATT (*Aylesbury*): I am afraid that I cannot accept Dr. Hinton's view. Professor Hamilton was discussing the assessment of the mental state of the patient by physiological functions. What has just been discussed is actually measuring the physiological functions— quite a different matter and, of course, much simpler.

DEREK RICHTER: Dr. Steinberg mentioned the use in some experiments of drugs which can affect the temperature of small animals such as rats and mice. We have found that the hypothermic effect of barbiturates or phenothiazines can have quite an appreciable effect on the behaviour of animals and I wonder if in Dr. Steinberg's experiments the temperature was controlled.

T. S. DAVIES (*Cwmbran, Mon.*): There is one fact which I think should be stressed. This is the effect of the genetic pattern of the patient and the natural passage of time in the case of any long drawn out illness. The genetic background is obviously important in considering the way a patient will respond to a drug and yet we have heard no mention of it.

HANNAH STEINBERG: May I deal with some of the points raised? In answer to Dr. Richter's question about temperature, indeed it is very necessary to keep it constant, and we use a thermostat to keep it at 70–72°F. At higher temperatures barbiturates in particular seem to be more active (cf. Keplinger, Lanier and Deichmann[2]).

As for Dr. Oswald's report about long-term effects, I should also like to underline what Dr. Himwich said in the discussion. There are certainly differences between giving drugs to patients and giving them to normal people. The same dose of the same drug may " normalize " the behaviour of a patient, but may make the behaviour of a normal patient abnormal and this may be undesirable. Marked differences in the effects of drugs according to what one might call the behavioural base-line of the subjects can also be demonstrated in animals, as I have described in my paper (p. 27). However, I agree with Dr. Oswald that administration of a drug can sometimes have effects long after it has apparently been completely removed from the body.

Dr. Russell Barton objected to the use of " fear " in interpreting the results of animal experiments. Naturally this is an inference from the observed behaviour, but so it is too when we infer fear in man. A man can talk about his subjective experiences, but this is only one aspect of his observable behaviour and we look for agreement with other aspects, like avoiding the situation, physiological signs and so on, in making the inference. Animals cannot talk, but we can, as in man, compare the results of procedures which approach the problem from different angles as I showed when I referred to Miller's experiments on amylobarbitone (p. 26). When the results correlate they reinforce the interpretation. In studying fear in animals one can make use of stimuli which are noxious to them, like electric shocks, as one can in studying fear in man. Such experiments do not stand or fall by the use of words like " fear "; one can discuss them in other terms like " avoidance behaviour " instead.

Dr. Smythies asked about rope climbing and the depression of muscle activity. It seems to me very possible that in some of the experiments using such techniques animals were made ataxic or otherwise impaired in their muscle activity by the drug. In such cases results showing worse performance in tests of rope climbing to obtain food may have to be interpreted cautiously; and it might in any case be useful to measure other aspects of muscle activity, e.g. ataxia, separately and in ways which do not involve food rewards.

E

A. SUMMERFIELD: I should like to take up both Dr. Russell Barton's points.

First, I agree with what Dr. Steinberg has just said about using terms like " fear " and " anxiety " in explaining the results of these experiments on animals. There is no more difference in principle in doing this than talking about electrons and other atomic particles in physics. The test is in terms of prediction. Dr. Steinberg referred to different sorts of experiments both of her own and of Professor Neal Miller at Yale (p. 26). The results of these experiments could be interpreted in terms of anxiety or fear and the interpretations then used to predict the results of other different experiments.

The second point which follows on from this is to challenge the notion that there is something special about " subjective experience ". If one is talking about subjective experience one is relying in some way upon what a person says. This is only one way in which a person can behave and, in fact, we do not just rely upon what a person says. We certainly take into account other aspects of his behaviour. For example, a psychiatrist friend tells me that in interviewing he normally asks his depressed patients a series of direct questions, including " Have you ever thought of taking your own life? ". Some depressed patients would react by saying " Oh, no, Doctor! ", but they would shrink back in their chair away from him at the same time! His inference from this was, of course, that the patient *had* thought at some time of taking his own life. He did not rely upon the statement that the patient had made about his subjective experience.

M. HAMILTON: I think that there is some confusion about the meaning of words rather than the intent of what we are talking about in the discussion by Dr. Watts and Dr. Hinton.

Let us consider, for example, Dr. Oswald's paper. He used there a physiological measure to demonstrate the action of the drug. He was concerned solely to demonstrate that the drug, using this measure, had effects which transcend the period of its usage. He was not using this measure to determine whether it was hypnotic, whether in fact the patient was sleeping and as such subjectively felt he had slept. Nor was he measuring whether the sleep had the refreshing quality that normal sleep has. He was not concerned here primarily with the psychological effect but using the physiological measure as an index of drug activity. Now this in a sense is an extreme position. There is an opposite extreme in which one uses some physiological measure solely because it is considered to reflect the psychological state of the patient. The pulse rate will go up when we become anxious or tense or alarmed. If it can be shown that anxiety neurotics have a bigger response than normal individuals, and if it can be shown that a certain drug diminishes the response— normalizes it so to speak—then we conclude that the drug has an effect on the anxiety of the patient.

But the point I was making, and I must apologize to Dr. Watt if I did not make it clear because I entirely agree with him, is that we can use physiological measurements as an index of psychological changes only if we first prove that there is a relationship between the two. We must validate the measures. There seems to be a view at present that judgmental methods of assessing changes in patients, i.e. ratings, questionnaires, overall assessment, are in some way less scientific than physiological readings on gadgets. In fact, the most direct way of assessing the behaviour is to assess the behaviour, to use anything else is going one step away from behaviour. If we are going to use the other measurements we must prove that they are valid.

I. OSWALD: Following on what Dr. Himwich and Dr. Steinberg have said may I stress that the people used for the sedative study were normal or as normal as volunteers can ever be. There is no *a priori* reason to suppose that patients might show different reactions.

REFERENCES

1. TAKAHASHI, Y. and AKABANE, Y., *Arch. gen. Psychiat.* **3**, 674 (1960).
2. KEPLINGER, M. L., LANIER, G. E. and DEICHMANN, W. B., *Toxicol. appl. Pharmacol.* **1**, 156 (1959).

SESSION II

MAJOR TRANQUILLIZERS

Chairman: Professor W. M. MILLAR

CLINICAL USE OF THE PHENOTHIAZINES

JOHN DENHAM

Summary—Clinical use of the phenothiazines preceded the establishment of a scientific basis of drug treatment in psychiatry. As most drug treatment remains symptomatic the clinician depends on further scientific advances for an explanation of pharmacological action; this may produce a new aetiology and specific treatment. In the meantime the clinician depends on the phenothiazines for the suppression of symptom-complexes which cut across the major psychiatric disease entities. The phenothiazines control abnormal and excessive psychomotor activity in schizophrenia, manic-depressive psychosis and organic psychosis, they are active in anxiety and tension states, and are used in a large variety of conditions for anti-pruritic, anti-emetic and anti-parkinsonian activity.

Mode of administration and dosage follows traditional pharmacological lines, though occasionally heroic treatment is undertaken in resistant cases with high doses limited only by the appearance of toxic manifestations. The discontinuous method of treatment of schizophrenia with thioproperazine and the relationship to drug-induced parkinsonism is discussed. The importance and the hazards of maintenance therapy are mentioned.

The choice of individual phenothiazine compound depends largely on post-graduate education supplied by the drug-houses for the clinicians, while the latter disseminate their personal preferences. The results of clinical trials arrive too late to influence clinical choice of drugs. Trials assist materially with the raising of morale of chronic patients and staff, but add little to the treatment of recent patients. These are usually sophisticated and prefer insight-giving therapy, and express widely held ambivalence towards drugs acting on the central nervous system.

Résumé—L'emploi clinique des phénothiazines a précédé l'établissement d'une base scientifique de la chimiothérapie en psychiatrie. Etant donné que la plupart des traitements médicamenteux restent symptomatiques, le clinicien dépend d'autres progrés scientifiques pour une explication de leur action pharmacologique; ceci peut permettre de trouver une nouvelle étiologie et un traitement spécifique. Entre-temps, le clinicien est tributaire des phénothiazines pour la suppression des complexes de troubles qui recoupent la plupart des entités des affections psychiatriques. Les phénothiazines contrôlent l'activité psychomotrice excessive dans la schizophrénie, la psychose maniaque dépressive et les psychoses organiques. Elles sont efficaces dans les états d'anxiété et de tension et sont utilisées dans de nombreux états patho-logiques pour leur effet antiprurigineux, antiémétique et anti-parkinsonien.

Le mode d'administration et la posologie suivent les schémas pharmacologiques traditionnels bien qu'occasionnellement dans les cas résistants, on entreprenne un traitement " héroïque " avec des doses élevées, limitées seulement par l'apparition de manifestations toxiques. Le méthode thérapeutique discontinue de la schizo-phrénie avec la thiopropérazine et la relation avec le parkinsonisme provoqué médicamenteusement sont discutées. On mentionne également l'importance et les aléas de la thérapie continue.

Le choix d'un dérivé particulier de la phénothiazine dépend dans une large mesure des cours de perfectionnement offerts par les maisons pharmaceutiques pour les cliniciens qui peuvent propager leurs préférences personnelles. Les résultats des études cliniques arrivent trop tard pour influencer le choix clinique des médicaments.

Les tests contribuent grandement à relever le moral des malades chroniques et du personnel mais n'apportent que peu de choses au traitement des cas récents. Ils sont généralement plus compliqués et préfèrent un traitement qui les aide à voir leurs problèmes; en outre ils se comportent d'une manière ambivalente à l'égard des médicaments agissant sur le systéme nerveux central.

Zusammenfassung—Die klinische Verwendung von Phenothiazinen ging der Schaffung einer wissenschaftlichen Grundlage für die Psychopharmakotherapie voraus. Da die medikamentöse Behandlung psychischer Leiden meist nur symptomatischer Art ist, bedarf der Kliniker weiterer wissenschaftlicher Fortschritte, um die pharmakologische Wirkung erklären zu können; möglicherweise wirft weitere Forschungsarbeit auch ein neues Licht auf die Ätiologie und führt zu spezifischer Therapie. Bis dahin ist der Kliniker für die Beseitigung von Symptomenkomplexen, die in allen Hauptkategorien psychischer Erkrankungen anzutreffen sind, auf die Phenothiazine angewiesen. Die Phenothiazine dämpfen übermässige psychomotorische Aktivität bei Schizophrenie, Zyklothymie und organisch bedingten Psychosen; sie beeinflussen Angst- und Spannungszustände und werden ihrer antipruritischen, antiemetischen und Antiparkinson-Wirkung wegen bei einer grossen Zahl verschiedenartiger Krankheitsbilder verwendet.

Dosierung und Verabreichungsweise folgen klassischen pharmakologischen Richtlinien, wenn auch gelegentlich in refranktären Fällen zu drastischer Behandlung gegriffen wird, wobei die Dosishöhe nur durch das Auftreten von Toxizitätszeichen begrenzt wird. Die Intervallbehandlung der Schizophrenie mit Thioporperazin und der Zusammenhang mit medikamentös induziertem Parkinsonismus wird diskutiert. Die Bedeutung und die Risiken der Erhaltungstherapie werden erwähnt.

Die Wahl eines bestimmten Phenothiazinderivats hängt einerseits von den Informationen ab, die die Herstellerfirmen geben, andererseits von der persönlichen Vorliebe des Klinikers für das eine oder andere Präparat. Die Ergebnisse klinischer Untersuchungen kommen zu spät, um einen Einfluss auf diese Wahl auszuüben. Die klinische Prüfung neuer Präparate trägt wesentlich zur Stimmungshebung der Chronischkranken bei, ist aber für die Behandlung frischer Fälle von geringer Bedeutung, da diese meist die weitverbreitete Skepsis gegenüber Medikamenten, die das ZNS beeinflussen, teilen.

THE clinical use of the phenothiazines preceded the establishment of a scientific basis. For a considerable time animal experiments and clinical observations, often unrelated, provided the only available knowledge. To the clinician every single patient presents a fresh scientific experiment, rarely repeatable, defying quantification through abundance of variables. The clinician's efforts tend to be described as artistic rather than scientific, and yet significant advances in medicine are more often based on clinical observations than laboratory techniques.

The clinical trial has been introduced by the clinicians as a protest or apology and has swelled the volumes of medical literature. It is significant that a clinical trial in a chronic psychiatric ward increases morale and interest to the great benefit of the patients while in the treatment of the acute patients it may produce disruption.

In describing the use of the phenothiazines mention should be made of indications, mode of administration, dosage in the acute and maintenance treatment, sensitivity, tolerance and habituation, absorption and excretion, duration of action, hangover and rebound, complications, side effects and toxicity, going far beyond the scope of this paper. Furthermore, it is not proposed to give a review of the many hundred papers written on the subject but to underline such observations as may assist our understanding of the usage of the phenothiazines.

The phenothiazines are used to suppress symptoms, they have no direct effect on any psychiatric disease process. Indications for use are therefore directed towards symptoms or rather symptom-complexes only. In self-limiting disorders they may accelerate recovery, in progressive conditions they may retard progression and assist in rehabilitation. The foremost indication for their use is in disturbances of psychomotor behaviour in schizophrenia, the agitation and over-activity in affective disorders, and the motor-restlessness of the organic psychoses. Their initial action in these conditions is to divorce pathologic process from the effector organ. Without materially altering the psychiatric disorder normalization of behaviour is obtained. The usefulness of the less potent phenothiazines in states of anxiety may also be due to their diminution of autonomic reaction to anxiety. It is a debatable assumption that the autonomic and motor symptoms act like a feedback in the maintenance of psychiatric disorders which can be ameliorated by the interruption of the feedback-system.

A psycho-corrective action has been attributed to some phenothiazines which are useful in suppression of endo-psychic symptoms like hallucinations, delusions, morbid fears and impulses. A more articulate patient may be able to describe the disappearance of auditory hallucinations as they change during treatment from voices specifically directed towards himself from an outside agency, to voices heard inside his head, to thoughts being repeated and directed, and rarely to insight into the pathological origin of the auditory hallucinations.

Most phenothiazines have some degree of sedative action and potentiate the action of other sedatives and hypnotics. This led to the introduction of chlorpromazine into psychiatry. From its original use in the lytic cocktail it was found effective as a potentiator of pentothal in the control of turbulent patients in French casualty departments. Its use, together with amylobarbitone sodium, allowed for safer and more effective prolonged narcosis.[1]

In the treatment of schizophrenia, chlorpromazine entered the field at the same time as reserpine. In the hebephrenic the first and more spectacular results were achieved. Effectiveness was, however, limited to control of abnormal behaviour without alteration of the affective blunting and thought-disorder. More promising results are achieved in paranoid schizophrenia and other paranoid states where preservation of personality is more complete and symptom-suppression apparently more effective. The patients' failure to achieve insight enough to continue medication leads to frequent recurrences.

The failure of chlorpromazine to influence the bulk of chronic schizo-phrenic patients, the so-called deteriorated cases or états vegetatives, led to the search for more potent compounds. It was soon recognized that the introduction of the piperazine side-chain increased potency in the treatment of schizophrenia together with an increased tendency to produce extra-pyramidal side effects, and a reduction of sedative action. This extended their range of usefulness in the treatment of schizophrenia to the catatonic deteriorated chronic patients. Schizophrenic deterioration was proved to be a reversible process and not a progressive dementia.

The value of the phenothiazines in the treatment of the recent schizo-phrenic and the acutely relapsing case is undisputed. With effective dosage remissions are obtainable within 10 days to 3 weeks. Affective blunting is avoided. Often, remission is preceded by a short period of depression followed by a most welcome state of elation. This tendency towards manic-depressive mood-swings has been noted particularly in follow-up of juvenile schizophrenics. It may respond to antidepressant medication, rehabilitative and re-educative measures, and sometimes to psychotherapeutic interven-tions. Prolonged follow-up seems to confound those who state that the outcome of schizophrenia after five years is the same irrespective of treatment or rehabilitation.

In cases of mania the effectiveness of a phenothiazine compound is pro-portional to its activity in schizophrenia. Symptom suppression is rapid and effective; more so than with lithium carbonate and about equal to halo-peridol. Treatment may have to be continued until spontaneous remission occurs but with the addition of electroconvulsive therapy the attack can be cut short. Excessive medication leads to depression less frequently than with haloperidol.

The ability to control the restlessness and agitation in depressive states led to the recognition of two distinct components in depressive illnesses: the one being depression and retardation, the other consisting of anxiety and agitation. In the search for compounds acting in both, the so-called biphasic antidepressants were introduced. Levomepromazine is claimed to be the only antidepressant phenothiazine. Prochlorperazine has specific usefulness in the treatment of depressions with tinnitus.

Motor restlessness in mental defectives, and in toxic and organic psychosis is often well controlled by phenothiazines. Restlessness in the elderly responds well to the phenothiazines and promazine enjoys great popularity because of the claim of safety. Promethazine has been found to be equally safe and is effective in the elderly both as a diurnal sedative and as a hypnotic. Chlor-promazine although eminently effective as a hypnotic has a tendency to produce confusion and lower the blood pressure dangerously in the hyper-tensive, and thioridazine has tended to replace it.

In childhood the phenothiazines can be used in spite of the readiness with which they produce extrapyramidal symptoms. They will arrest progression of schizophrenia, control hyperkinesis, and improve general health but have little effect in the autistic child. Anxiety states in the young respond to the phenothiazines though they should be avoided as they produce dullness and impair intellectual functioning.

A number of phenothiazines, especially promethazine and chlorpromazine have been widely used in non-psychiatric conditions as antipruritics, antiemetics, as antiparkinsonian drugs, as adjuvants in anaesthesia and in the treatment of intractable pain. Chlorpromazine is unique amongst the phenothiazines in the ability to improve appetite and reverse weight-loss. Prochlorperazine enjoys a high reputation as an antiemetic in obstetrics, while levomepromazine is a favourite amongst surgeons. Chlorpromazine is widely used in the treatment of asthma and is especially effective in preventing nocturnal attacks if taken in the evening.

A curious indication is presented by the usefulness of the more toxic phenothiazines in the control of ataxia, chorea and athetosis. Thiopropazate and thioproperazine have been effective in Huntington's chorea. The propensity to increase muscular tone and so effect isotonic contraction perhaps counterbalances the disturbed isometric contractions in these conditions.

Considerable contradictions exist about the use of low dosage trifluoperazine, prochlorperazine and perphenazine in anxiety and tension states. Efficient sales promotion and prescribing habits may account for their widespread use.

It is next to impossible to give indications objectively for the individual phenothiazines. Every doctor should know one or two compounds well, use them effectively and not change them too frequently. The careful doctor will choose a safe compound and be content with somewhat delayed results. In an efficient hospital setting the drug with higher potency and greater toxicity can be selected. However, claims of safety accepted complacently have been known to lead to disasters.

In psychiatry it is particularly important to keep prescription and treatment instructions simple and clear. Multiple prescriptions and frequent changes only confuse the patient and all those around him. Examples could be cited of patients receiving 6–8 drugs at once who only improved when all were discontinued. In this country, oral administration in tablet form is preferred, the liquid form is reserved for those who find it difficult, or refuse to swallow tablets. Injection increases the effectiveness of phenothiazines 5 to 10 times and reduces the delay in onset of action to a minimum.

An adequate dose of chlorpromazine may take from 1 to 2 weeks to be effective, for prochlorperazine this would be 10 days, for trifluoperazine 3 and thioproperazine 1 to 2 days. Remarkably little work has been done in the field of absorption, blood levels and tissue distribution of the phenothiazines.

The amounts of phenothiazines prescribed commonly vary only within narrow limits. A few have been used with ingenuity and daring in their dosage schemes. Chlorpromazine and thioridazine have been given in doses up to 4000 mg daily mainly in the United States. Several psychiatrists have raised the daily amount until toxic symptoms became apparent. It is usually the appearance of severe Parkinsonism that limits further increases. Treatment has to be interrupted until side effects disappear. This led Delay to introduce discontinuous treatment of schizophrenics, mainly with thioproperazine.[2] In this form of treatment thioproperazine is given initially in a dosage of 5 mg 8 hourly on the first day and increased daily by 5 mg until extrapyramidal symptoms appear. The dosage is then maintained at that level for 5 days and discontinued abruptly. During the following two days most of the side effects disappear and psychiatric improvement, if any, is most noticeable. Further courses of treatment can be given if need be, starting with the maximum dose or just below. As improvement eventually becomes established the patients become more sensitive to the drug, an observation almost unique with central acting drugs. During this treatment hallucinations disappear at an early stage, affective blunting may turn into depression with suicidal tendencies, to be followed by elation when treatment has been interrupted. This discontinuous form of treatment is especially effective in the young and recent schizophrenic and also may be used in the severely retarded and apathetic patient. In the latter group florid symptoms may be re-awakened during the course of treatment and be suppressed later. The results, if perhaps not numerically superior, are certainly qualitatively more marked than those with normal continuous therapy.[3] Lately we have used trifluoperazine in a similar manner with greater safety and good results.

This type of discontinuous treatment has raised a number of interesting questions. The one usually asked when psychiatric claims are made is how much improvement is due to the need for intensive medical and nursing care. This form of treatment certainly arouses great interest among staff who normally become disinterested with every-day dosage schemes. During treatment distonic attacks occur that are alarming and painful for the patients. These attacks—often called excitomotor attacks—are provoked by some minor stress or are induced by observing similar attacks in other patients. They respond to medication but also to suggestion and command. This led Delay and Deniker to formulate a theory of hysteria.[4] We have tried to utilize the increased suggestibility during treatment to dislodge some of the firmly fixed delusions. When parkinsonism appears, a conflict about the administration or withholding of anti-parkinsonian agents occurs, together with the question about any possible improvement being related to the presence of extrapyramidal symptoms. Most will regard those symptoms as toxic and will avoid, suppress and prevent them, while some will regard them as indicators of an effective dose level. Finally complications can appear suddenly during discontinuous treatment; they may be severe and have been known to be fatal. Theoretical implications raised by this form of treatment have not been answered.[4] We have investigated certain physiological reactions known to be abnormal in schizophrenia such as sensitivity to epinephrine, mecholyl, insulin and lysergic acid, and found that successful treatment tends to increase sensitivity reactions towards a normal level.[5]

Long-term maintenance treatment with phenothiazines is of great importance in schizophrenia. Generally, one can say that dosage should be raised as rapidly as possible until symptoms are suppressed and then reduced until a minimum is reached that will keep symptoms in abeyance. It is unwise to change to a different drug at this stage. If the minimum dose induces extrapyramidal symptoms an anti-parkinsonian agent should be given. We prescribe orphenadrine when the patient requires a degree of stimulation and phenergen if sedation is needed.

Minor improvement may continue during maintenance therapy and dosage can then be reduced further. An indication for further reduction is the appearance of minor side effects like drowsiness and tremor, again suggesting that the improving patient becomes more sensitive to the drug. In such cases chlorpromazine can be replaced by thioridazine at the same dose level. During periods of stress or anxiety the patients will require increased amounts to preserve their stability. In spite of the simplicity of treatment, instruction defaults are frequent and frustrating. The most successful patients were those who received their supply monthly by post.

Phenothiazines have been given to individual patients continuously for several years without any ill effect. Danish workers described 8 cases with persistent, involuntary mouth, neck and shoulder movements after maintenance dosage on perphenazine and ECT.[6] All cases were past middle age and a degenerative lesion could not be excluded. I saw a similar case after thioproperazine lasting 8 months before gradual disappearance of the most marked choreiform movements of mouth, head and shoulders. These were aggravated by the most minor sensory stimulation, disappeared during work and during sleep. Lately a purple discoloration of the skin has been observed after prolonged administration of chlorpromazine and attributed to the adrenaline-chromatine mechanism.

REFERENCES

1. DENHAM, J., In *West-African Med. J.* (Special Number 1962).
2. DELAY, J., DENIKER, P., FOURMENT, J., GREEN, A. and ROPERT, M., *Ann. med.-psychol.* **115**, 510 (1957).
3. DENHAM, J., In *Extrapyramidal System and Neuroleptics*, p. 449, November, 1961.
4. DELAY, J. and DENIKER, P., *Canad. psychiat. Ass. J.* **3**, 132 (1958).
5. DENHAM, J. and CARRICK, D. J. E. L., *J. ment. Sci.* **107**, 326 (1961).
6. UHRBRAND, L. and FAURBYE, A., *Psychopharmacologia (Berl.)* **1**, 408 (1960).

MODE OF ACTION OF THE PHENOTHIAZINES

Derek Richter

Summary—The phenothiazines are, *in vitro*, powerful metabolic blocking agents and they act in the respiratory chain at the flavoprotein level. However, it is doubtful if this is their main action *in vivo*, since the brain levels of ATP and creatine phosphate are relatively high after treatment with chlorpromazine whereas the reverse would be expected if the drug competed with flavine adenine dinucleotide, as has been suggested. In low doses chlorpromazine has been shown to accelerate the turnover rate of phospholipids *in vivo*. This effect is specific for the phospholipids of the brain and it is of particular interest since the phenothiazines are concentrated in the mitochondrial membranes of the nerve cells, which are rich in phospholipids. The phenothiazines have been shown to interfere with the transport of many metabolites in the brain. However, this action is not specific for the brain and, since it is shown also by other surface-active substances, it is difficult to relate this effect directly to the highly specific pharmacological action on the central nervous system. The psychotropically active phenothiazines, however, all have a central sympatholytic action: it has been suggested that this may be due to their interfering with the transport of biogenic amines from the point of synthesis to the storage sites or to the receptor sites in the brain.

Résumé—Les phénothiazines sont, *in vitro*, des agents puissants de blocage du métabolisme. Elles agissent sur la chaîne respiratoire au niveau des flavoprotéines. Cependant, il est douteux que cette action est de grande importance *in vivo*. Si les faits suggèrent que la concentration d'ATP et de phosphate de créatine est relativement élevée dans le cerveau après traitement à la chlorpromazine, on devrait s'attendre à la constatation inverse si le médicament entrait en compétition avec la flavine-adénine-dinucléotide, comme on l'a avancé. Il a toutefois été démontré qu'à doses faibles, la chlorpromazine accélérait le métabolisme des phospholipides. Ce phénomène était spécifique pour les phospholipides du cerveau. Il s'agit là de faits d'un intérêt particulier car les phénothiazines sont concentrées dans les membranes mitochondriales des cellules nerveuses, ces dernières riches en phospholipides. Les phénothiazines peuvent interférer avec le transport de nombreux métabolites dans le cerveau. Cette action n'est pourtant pas particulière au niveau cérébral et, comme on l'a vu pour d'autres agents surfactifs, il est difficile d'établir une relation directe entre l'effet mentionné et l'action pharmacologique très spécifique qui s'exerce sur le système nerveux central. Toutes les phénothiazines qu'avant l'action psychatropique ont un effet sympathicolytique central: l'hypothèse a été avancée que ceci pouvait être dû à l'interférence avec le transport des amines biogènes du lieu de leur synthèse aux dépôts ou aux récepteurs cérébraux.

Zusammenfassung—Die Phenothiazine wirken als starke Stoffwechselhemmer in die Atmungskette ein, und zwar auf der Flavoproteinstufe. Es ist allerdings zweifelhaft, ob dies für das *Invivo*-Verhalten von schwerer Bedeutung ist, da alle bekannten Anhaltspunkte darauf hindeuten, dass die ATP- und die Kreatinphosphat-Spiegel im Gehirn nach Behandlung mit Chlorpromazin verhältnismässig hoch sind, während das Gegenteil der Fall sein müsste, würde das Medikament sich dem Flavoadenindinukleotid gegenüber kompetitiv verhalten, wie man angenommen hatte. Es konnte indessen nachgewiesen werden, dass Chlorpromazin in niedrigen Dosen den Phospholipidstoffwechsel *in vivo* beschleunigt, und dies spezifisch im

Gehirn. Diese Feststellung ist von besonderem Interesse, da die Phenothiazine in den Mitochondrien der Nervenzellen konzentriert sind und diese reich an Phospholipiden sind. Die Phenothiazine können in den Transport vieler Metaboliten im Gehirn eingreifen. Allerdings ist diese Wirkung nicht hirnspezifisch, und, wie aus den Beobachtungen mit anderen oberflächenaktiven Substanzen hervorgeht, ist es schwierig, diesen Effekt mit der hochgradig spezifischen pharmakologischen Wirkung auf das ZNS in direkte Beziehung zu setzen. Immerhin haben alle Phenothiazine für die Psychopharmaleotherapie eine zentrale sympathicolytische Wirkung. Es ist die Hypothese aufgestellt worden, dies könnte darauf zurückzuführen sein, dass sie in den Transport körpereigener Amine vom Punkt ihrer Entstehung zum Ort ihrer Lagerung oder den zerebralen Rezeptoren eingreifen.

INFORMATION about the metabolic actions of the phenothiazines can be useful in extending our understanding of the way in which they work and in enabling us to avoid any dangers that may be associated with their use. It can also be helpful in planning the development of new and more effective drugs for use in the treatment of nervous and mental disorders.

Some of the properties of the phenothiazines can be inferred at once from their chemical structure. The psychotropically active compounds, such as chlorpromazine, have a hydrocarbon side-chain attached to a phenothiazine nucleus similar to that in methylene blue. It can be seen that they are substances of the kind that are soluble in lipid-solvents and that tend to attach themselves to lipid surfaces. The phenothiazine drugs resemble the biogenic amines in having an aromatic nucleus attached by a carbon chain to a basic amino group. We can therefore expect them to have some affinity for the amine receptor sites. It may be noted further that in the general shape of the molecule the phenothiazine drugs bear a superficial resemblance to riboflavin, which also has a 3-ring system attached to a carbon side-chain.

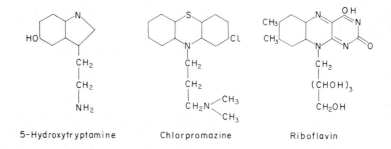

5-Hydroxytryptamine   Chlorpromazine   Riboflavin

FIG. 1.   Structural formulae of 5-hydroxytryptamine, chlorpromazine and riboflavin.

BIOCHEMICAL ACTIONS OF THE PHENOTHIAZINES

The actions of the psychotropically active phenothiazines can be considered at a number of different levels. At a molecular level we can study their metabolic effects, such as their interactions with enzymes and their biophysical actions in blocking the transport of metabolites through membranes. Information of this kind has proved especially valuable in the case of the anticholinesterases and monoamine oxidase inhibitors which produce many of their characteristic effects by their property of strongly inhibiting certain enzymes. At a higher organizational level we can study the pharmacological actions of drugs on individual organs and isolated functional systems. Finally, at the highest level, we can study their effects on the whole animal *in vivo*, investigating their metabolic and electrophysiological actions and their general effects on animal behaviour.

In the earlier studies of the actions of the phenothiazines on enzymes, tissue preparations were incubated with various concentrations of the drugs and a number of inhibitory effects were noted. It was found, for example, that 10^{-3} M chlorpromazine inhibited the respiration of brain slices by 90 per cent, owing apparently to inhibition of cytochrome oxidase. Chlorpromazine when incubated with brain slices also inhibited the ATP-ase system and uncoupled oxidative phosphorylation, causing a decrease in the ATP and creatine phosphate levels. But, a concentration of 10^{-3} M corresponds to a dose level of about 350 mg/kg, which is far above the range of therapeutic dose levels. At concentrations of the order of 10^{-5} M, corresponding to a dose level of 3·5 mg/kg, the respiration of brain slices was not significantly inhibited and oxidative phosphorylation was unimpaired. On the other hand some actions of the phenothiazine drugs were still observed at concentrations between 10^{-5} M and 10^{-6} M, which correspond more closely to dose levels at which the drugs are pharmacologically active in the body.

McIlwain and Greengard[1] found that chlorpromazine inhibited the respiration of electrically stimulated brain slices at concentrations down to 5×10^{-6} M. Attempts to locate more precisely the point of action of chlorpromazine in the electron transport chain gave evidence that it acts at more than one point but the most sensitive is the oxidation of DPNH by flavoprotein, which is one of the main sites of oxidative phosphorylation.[2] In agreement with this view Löw[3] showed that the phenothiazine drugs interfere specifically with the functions of the flavin of the mitochondrial flavoprotein system in its role as a phosphate carrier: the inhibitory action of phenothiazines on the mitochondrial ATP-ase is relieved by the addition of flavin adenine dinucleotide (FAD). Independent evidence that chlorpromazine can act as a flavin antagonist was given by the work of Yagi, Nagatsu and Ozawa[4] who showed that chlorpromazine competes with FAD for the protein of D-amino acid oxidase. These experiments indicate that the phenothiazines must be classed as powerful metabolic blocking agents and that their point of action in the respiratory chain is mainly at the flavoprotein level. But, it does not follow that this is the mechanism by which they act *in vivo* in producing their pharmacological effects. If the phenothiazines acted *in vivo* by inhibiting respiration one would expect to find reduced levels of high-energy phosphate esters in the brain. However, it has been shown that the levels of ATP and creatine phosphate in the brain are relatively high after treatment with chlorpromazine in animals rapidly killed by immersion in liquid air.[5] It would appear therefore that the respiratory system and oxidative phosphorylation are not primarily concerned in the pharmacological actions of these drugs.

In animals killed by decapitation, the ATP content of the brain quickly falls after death but it was found by Weiner and Huls[5] that the post mortem disappearance of ATP was reduced in animals that had been treated with chlorpromazine. This showed that chlorpromazine can depress the utilization of ATP and suggests that it may have an inhibitory action *in vivo* on anabolic reactions which utilize high-energy phosphate bonds. Evidenc: of an action of this kind was obtained by Ansell and Dohmen[6], who showed that chlorpromazine (5 mg/kg) inhibited the incorporation of labelled phosphate into the phospholipids of the rat brain. Magee, Berry and Rossiter[7] observed a similar inhibitory effect on the level of labelled phosphate of phospholipids in brain slices *in vitro* at concentrations down to 10^{-3} M chlorpromazine, but they found an *increased* labelled phosphate level with lower concentrations of the drug. This effect of chlorpromazine in accelerating the turnover rate of phospholipids was found also by Grossi, Paoletti and Paoletti[8] in studies of the incorporation of ^{14}C-acetate into the phospholipids of the rat brain *in vivo*. The effect was observed with doses down to 3·5 mg/kg in young animals, and they showed that it is specific for the phospholipids of the brain: the turnover of the liver phospholipids was not affected by chlorpromazine at the concentration used. The point of action of chlorpromazine in influencing phospholipid metabolism is apparently the enzyme phosphorylcholine cytidyl transferase.[9]

Some of the metabolic actions of chlorpromazine *in vivo* are due to an increase in the level of plasma corticosteroids resulting from stimulation of the pituitary-adrenal system.[10] There is an associated increase in the level of plasma free fatty acids, which accumulate in the liver as triglycerides. Chlorpromazine commonly produces an increase in weight in human subjects when administered for a long period and it has been shown to exert a mild diabetogenic action in raising the fasting blood sugar level and decreasing glucose tolerance in 30 per cent of subjects.[11] It would appear that chlorpromazine influences a number of different enzyme systems and produces a profound overall effect on the metabolism of the body. It remains doubtful to what extent these metabolic effects are responsible for the main central actions of the drug.

THE FATE OF PHENOTHIAZINES IN THE BODY

Another approach to the study of the actions of the phenothiazines is to consider the question of what happens to them when they are administered *in vivo*. Gothelf and Karczmar[12] studied the distribution of chlorpromazine in the organs of the cat after administration by intravenous injection. They found that the drug shifted rapidly from the blood into the tissues and the highest level was at first in the lung. After 60 min the concentration was about equally high in lung, liver and brain, and considerably lower in the other organs of the body. If we consider a drug's-eye-view of the body it is understandable that a lipid-soluble molecule such as that of chlorpromazine would tend to adhere to the lipid surfaces of the capillaries and would accumulate at first in the large vascular bed of the lung. Thereafter it is reasonable that it should accumulate in organs such as the brain and liver which are both vascular and have a relatively high lipid content. It is noteworthy that, at later times, there was found to be a significant accumulation of the drug in the body fat. The levels in the brain and other organs were still relatively high at 48 hr after administration. There were no very large differences in content in different parts of the brain.

Evidence of the distribution of phenothiazines in nervous tissues was obtained by Murray and Peterson[13] who studied the localization of chlorpromazine in tissue cultures of nerve cells. They found, by fluorescence microscopy, that chlorpromazine was concentrated in the mitochondrial zone of the nerve cell bodies: it was also bound, less strongly, to the myelin. The mitochondrial membranes are rich in phospholipids and Roizin[14] showed by electron micrography, that prochlorperazine at doses down to 5 mg/kg causes a reversible alteration of the structure of brain and liver mitochondria, with a partial disintegration of the limiting membranes. These observations suggest that the pharmacological actions of the phenothiazines may be related to their tendency to accumulate at membrane surfaces in the cell.

The oxidation of chlorpromazine to the sulphoxide in the body leads to the final elimination of the drug.[15]

THE EFFECT OF PHENOTHIAZINES ON THE TRANSPORT OF METABOLITES

Several lines of investigation have given evidence of a blocking action of phenothiazines on the transport of metabolites in the tissues. Ernsting *et al.*[16] found that chlorpromazine (5×10^{-4} M) decreased the uptake of amino acids from the suspending medium into brain slices incubated *in vitro*. In similar experiments with brain slices it has been shown that 10^{-6} M chlorpromazine blocks the uptake of tritium-labelled noradrenaline.[17] Quadbeck[18] observed that doses of the order of 5 mg/kg of chlorpromazine affect the transport of labelled Na^+, phosphate and glucose into the mouse brain *in vivo*: it also blocks the uptake into the hypothalamus *in vivo* of labelled noradrenaline.[19] As might be expected from their tendency to accumulate at surface membranes, the phenothiazines are clearly active in

F

blocking the transport of metabolites but this action is unspecific since it is shown also by other surface-active substances and it occurs in tissues other than brain. It is difficult, therefore, to relate this effect directly to the highly specific pharmacological actions of the phenothiazines in the central nervous system.

THE TRANQUILLIZING ACTION OF THE PHENOTHIAZINES

In seeking a basis for the characteristic tranquillizing action of the phenothiazines it is relevant that they have been shown to exert a central sympatholytic action: in other words, they block the alerting effect of the biogenic amines in the brain.[20] In agreement with this view it has been shown that at a dose level of 1–3 mg/kg most of the psychotropic phenothiazines reverse the alerting action of amphetamine on the electrical activity of the rabbit brain.[21] Pletscher [22] has suggested that the sympatholytic action of the phenothiazines may be due to their interfering with the transport of biogenic amines from the point of synthesis to the storage sites or to the receptor sites in the brain and this is supported by the observation that chlorpromazine prevents the accumulation of serotonin in the brains of mice pretreated with monoamine oxidase inhibitors.[23] However, in a study of the properties of twenty-six different phenothiazines and related compounds, Steiner, Bost and Himwich[21] concluded that sympatholytic activity does not run parallel to sedative action in the phenothiazines. It would appear that other factors are also concerned in the tranquillizing action of these drugs.

In a study of the actions of phenothiazines in different animal species Brodie, Bogdanski and Bonomi[24] found that chlorpromazine has relatively little activity in submammalian species: a dose level giving 5 mg/kg chlorpromazine in the brain causes profound sedation in the rat, but doses 10 times as great in the pigeon and 50 times as great in frog and fish produce relatively little effect. The sedative action of the phenothiazines thus appears to depend to a considerable extent on structural or metabolic factors peculiar to the mammalian brain.

There is considerable evidence that the primary action of the phenothiazines is mainly at a subcortical level. Thus, the effect of chlorpromazine in preventing the spread of activation in the cortex of the cat brain depends on an action at the level of the brain stem reticular formation.[20, 25] In a study of the responses recorded by microelectrodes implanted in different areas of the cat brain, Valdman[26] showed that chlorpromazine reduces the spontaneous electrical activity of reticular neurones but the sensitivity to chlorpromazine varies greatly at different levels and also in different morphological structures in the brain stem.

It is clear that the phenothiazines have a number of biochemical and biophysical actions in influencing the activity of enzymes and the transport of metabolites in the cell but their characteristic action as tranquillizers apparently results from a complex interaction of biochemical, biophysical and morphological factors operating in subcortical regions of the mammalian brain.

REFERENCES

1. McIlwain, H. and Greengard, O., *J. Neurochem.* **1**, 348 (1957).
2. Dawkins, M. J. R., Judah, J. D. and Rees, K. R., *Biochem. J.* **73**, 16 (1959).
3. Löw, H., *Biochem. biophys. Acta (Amst.)* **32**, 11 (1959).
4. Yagi, K., Nagatsu, T. and Ozawa, T., *Nature (Lond.)* **177**, 891 (1956).
5. Weiner, N. and Huls, H. N., *J. Neurochem.* **7**, 180 (1961).
6. Ansell, G. B. and Dohmen, H., *J. Neurochem.* **1**, 150 (1956).
7. Magee, W. L., Berry, J. F. and Rossiter, R. J., *Biochem. biophys. Acta (Amst.)* **21**, 408 (1956).
8. Grossi, E., Paoletti, P. and Paoletti, R., *J. Neurochem.* **6**, 73 (1960).
9. Ansell, G. B. and Marshall, E. F., *J. Neurochem.* **10**, 875 and 883 (1963).
10. Paoletti, R. and Vertua, R., In *Comparative Neurochemistry*, p. 413, Ed. Richter, D., Pergamon Press, Oxford 1964.
11. Amdisen, A., Personal communication from Risskov Hospital, Aarhus, Denmark 1964.
12. Gothelf, B. and Karczmar, A. G., *Int. J. Neuropharmacol.* **2**, 39 (1963).
13. Murray, M. R. and Peterson, E. R., In *Comparative Neurochemistry*, p. 451, Ed. Richter, D., Pergamon Press, Oxford 1964.
14. Roizin, L., Kaufman, M., Bollard, B., Sabia, R. and Horwitz, W., *Psychopharmacol. Serv. Cent. Bull.* **2**, 81 (1962).
15. Salzman, N. P. and Brodie, B. B., *J. Pharmacol. Exp. Therap.* **118**, 46 (1956).
16. Ernsting, M. J. E., Kafoe, W. F., Nauta, W. Th., Oosterhuis, H. K. and DeWaart, C., *J. Neurochem.* **5**, 121 (1960).
17. Dengler, H. J., Spiegel, H. E. and Titus, E. O., *Nature (Lond.)* **191**, 816 (1961).
18. Quadbeck, G., *Proc. 4th Meeting Collegium Internationale Neuro-Psychopharmacologicum*, Birmingham 1964.
19. Weil-Malherbe, H., Whitby, L. G. and Axelrod, J., *J. Neurochem.* **8**, 55 (1961).
20. Bradley, P. B. and Hance, A. J., *Electroenceph. clin. Neurophysiol.* **9**, 191 (1957).
21. Steiner, W. G., Bost, K. and Himwich, H. E., *Int. J. Neuropharmacol.* **2**, 327 (1963).
22. Pletscher, A., *Proc. 4th Meeting Collegium Internationale Neuro-Psychopharmacologicum*, Birmingham, 1964.
23. Bartlet, A. L., *J. Physiol. (Lond.)* **165**, 25P (1963).
24. Brodie, B. B., Bogdanski, D. F. and Bonomi, L., In *Comparative Neurochemistry*, p. 367, Ed. Richter, D., Pergamon Press, Oxford 1964.
25. Anokhin, P., In *Biogenic Amines*, p. 223, Eds Himwich, H. E. and Himwich, W. A., Elsevier, Amsterdam 1964.
26. Valdman, A. N., *Int. J. Neuropharmacol.* **1**, 97 (1962).

STRUCTURE FUNCTIONAL RELATIONSHIPS
WITHIN THE PHENOTHIAZINE CLASS

PETER SAINSBURY

Summary—Structure functional relationships within the phenothiazine class of compounds is reviewed. Various substitutions at two positions in the basic phenothiazine ring can produce variations in both pharmacological activity and clinical side effects. Unfortunately similar useful correlations are not seen in the majority of studies in the clinic.

Résumé—Les rapports existant entre structure chimique et action pharmacodynamique sont passés en revue en ce qui concerne les phénothiazines. Différentes substitutions à deux endroits différents du noyau phénothiazinique peuvent se traduire par des variations dans l'action pharmacologique et les effets secondaires observés en clinique. Il faut regretter que d'utiles corrélations de ce genre soient absentes de la plupart des publications d'ordre clinique.

Zusammenfassung—Es werden strukturell-funktionelle Zusammenhänge innerhalb der Phenothiazingruppe besprochen. Verschiedene Substitutionen in zwei Positionen des ursprünglichen Phenothiazinringes können Variationen der pharmakologischen Wirkung wie der klinischen Nebenerscheinungen bewirken. Leider werden in der Mehrzahl der klinischen Arbeiten solche nützlichen Korrelationen nicht hergestellt.

THE phenothiazines we will discuss are those classified as the "major tranquillizers", and this description of them implies that the functions of most interest to us are those on behaviour and on the central nervous system. This at once brings us up against one of the difficulties of relating structure and function. The methods of the organic chemists are highly developed and their subject is very well ordered but the biologist's knowledge of the chemistry and physiology of the nervous system is far less sophisticated while the psychologist and psychiatrist have not even decided how best to describe their material and classify it, let alone measure the phenomena they study. The industrial chemist, the pharmacologist and the clinician are badly out of step; so while the chemist is able to modify a molecule in whatever way he is asked, we really have very little idea what to ask him to do with it, what additions to it to suggest which might help to elucidate the pharmacological chemistry of the nervous system, or to indicate what derivatives are likely to have salutory effects on behaviour. It is not surprising, therefore, that we are faced with an array of phenothiazines of all manner of shapes which hinder rather than help clinical research on the tranquillizers by

71

directing inquiries into yet further trials in which the patients' overall improvement on a new phenothiazine X is compared with that on Y. If we are not able to direct the industrial chemists' skill and energy to significant clinical and pharmacological problems we should not be surprised if, for want of better briefing, each pharmaceutical house introduces its own variation on the phenothiazine theme and then competes commercially for the enormous demand for tranquillizers. I am over-stating what, in fact, happens; nevertheless a problem of this kind does, I believe, exist. I also believe that there is a need to develop a more coherent organization by which industry, academic departments of pharmacology, and clinical research workers can collaborate more closely in the development, mode of action and clinical evaluation of new drugs. I hope to return to some aspects of this problem presently. Meanwhile I will discuss the structure of some of the phenothiazines we already have. Substitutions in the 2 and 10 positions of the nucleus are those which concern us, and they are shown as R_1 and R_2. It is variation in the chemical structure of these side-chains which affects the psychopharmacological functions of the tranquillizers. The parent substance, phenothiazine, which simply has H atoms at R_1 and R_2, made its debut in the pharmacopoeia many years ago as a rather unsuccessful anthelmintic; it had toxic effects on the blood and liver, a tendency which has been diminished but not eliminated in its derivatives.

The phenothiazine molecule reappeared in certain anti-histamine drugs of which promethazine is the most familiar example. In this compound R_1 is still an H atom, but R_2 has a side-chain with *two* carbon atoms in a straight line attached to the nitrogen of the nucleus but as Dr. Himwich has very nicely shown, the effects on the higher centres of the nervous system only appear in earnest when this side-chain consists of *three* carbon atoms in a row.[1] These central effects become less evident again if the chain of carbon atoms is increased to four. Nevertheless, promethazine with its short side-chain, has a sedative action, though resembling a barbiturate in this respect rather than a typical tranquillizer. A marked anti-histamine action of the phenothiazines apparently depends on an amino group being attached to an aliphatic chain in the β-position (see diagram).[2] The structure of one other derivative with a two carbon atom side-chain, diethazine, merits consideration, because of its marked anti-parkinsonian properties. As you know, a troublesome side effect of the tranquillizing phenothiazines is a tendency to induce extrapyramidal symptoms. But it seems that when the side-chain has two carbon atoms rather than three, and ends with a diethylamino group instead of a dimethylamino one, the action of the drug on the extrapyramidal system is reversed and its tranquillizing properties lost: a remarkable example of a small structural change having functional consequences of a marked and opposite kind. And to me this again emphasizes the enormous discrepancy between our ability to describe the niceties of

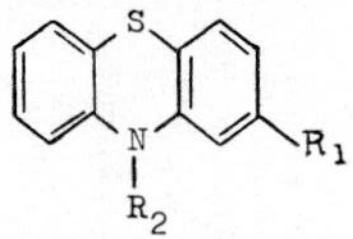

PHENOTHIAZINE. $(R_1 = H; R_2 = H)$

Derivative	R_1	R_2 (2 carbon side chain)	Comment	Potency as Tranquilliser Chlorpromazine = 1
Promethazine	H	$CH_2 - \underset{CH_3}{CH} - N(CH_3)_2$	Antihistaminic	0
Diethazine	H	$CH_2 - CH_2 - N(C_2H_5)_2$	Antiparkinsonian	0
		R_2 (3 carbon side chain)		
1. Aliphatic side chain:				
Promazine	H	$CH_2 - CH_2 - CH_2 - N(CH_3)_2$	Tranquilliser	½
Chlorpromazine	Cl	$CH_2 - CH_2 - CH_2 - N(CH_3)_2$	"	1
2. Piperidine side chain:				
Mepazine	H	CH_2 — (piperidine N-CH₃)	"	½
Thioridazine	SCH₃	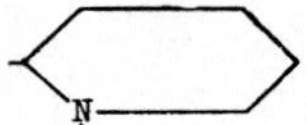 $CH_2 - CH_2$ — (piperidine N-CH₃)	"	1
3. Piperazine side chain:				
Prochlorperazine	Cl	$CH_2 - CH_2 - CH_2 - N$⟩N $- CH_3$ 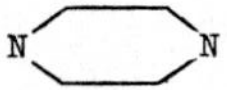	"	5
Trifluoperazine	CF₃	$CH_2 - CH_2 - CH_2 - N$⟩N $- CH_3$ 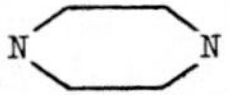	"	10

Fig. 1. The phenothiazine molecule and some of its important variants.

chemical structure and our inability to grasp the pharmacological import of them.

The phenothiazines which are effective tranquillizers in the sense that they calm over-active and distraught patients without necessarily inducing sleep or impairing consciousness are, then, those in which the R_1 side-chain has three carbon atoms in a row. Before attempting to subdivide this class structurally and functionally, I will enumerate those pharmacological actions which they have, to a greater or lesser extent in common. First, their other effects on behaviour. Animals, normally fierce, are tamed, and sham rage in cats is suppressed. Conditioned reflexes are abolished, though the response to the unconditioned stimulus remains. On the *motor* side they diminish restlessness, and this function may be mediated by a blocking effect on the descending pathways of the reticular formation. The response to *sensory* stimuli is diminished and this may lead to drowsiness, though the EEG pattern is not that which normally accompanies drowsiness. The activity of the reticular formation is depressed: it is thought that the collaterals entering the reticular formation from the sensory pathways are blocked, while activity in the main sensory tract to the cortex is preserved.[3, 4]

Next, a variety of functions mediated through the hypothalamus are depressed. The phenothiazines are adrenergic blocking agents, but they are also weakly anti-cholinergic. The net autonomic result is a tendency for many of them to induce hypotension and vasodilatation with consequent heat loss, though the latter is probably a consequence of suppression of the motor pathways mediating shivering. The activity of the pituitary is also affected through depression of centres in the hypothalamus. Finally, in the medullary region, the vomiting centre is depressed.

The tranquillizing derivatives of phenothiazine can be classified according to their chemical structure. Do these chemical groups also differentiate their pharmacological actions? And, more particularly, can the tranquillizers be distinguished by their effects on the behaviour of normal and of mentally ill people? Lastly, can their toxic effects be related to their differences in structure?

As I have already mentioned, the properties of the phenothiazine derivatives are mainly determined by the chemical substituents R_1 and R_2. The R_1 substitutions commonly made are the replacement of the H atom by a halogen, either chlorine or fluorine. Both increase the potency of the derivative, that is to say, they increase clinical effectiveness; they also alter the incidence and type of side effects—fluorine more so than chlorine. Fluorine in particular increases the incidence of extrapyramidal symptoms.

Tranquillizing phenothiazines are also formed by substitutions of R_2. These R_2 side-chains may be classified into three chemical groups:

(1) Derivatives with a three carbon atom aliphatic side-chain—a diethylaminopropyl group. Two widely used derivatives in which the R_2 side-chain

is of this structure are promazine in which R_1 is an H atom, and chlorpromazine in which R_1 is chlorine.

(2) Those with a piperidine side-chain. Mepazine with an H atom at R_1 is one example, thioridazine is another: the R_1 substitution in this derivative is not the usual halogen, but a SCH_3 group.

(3) Those with a piperazine side-chain. Prochlorperazine is one piperazine derivative—it has a chlorine atom at R_1. Another is trifluoperazine which only differs from prochlorperazine by having a carbon and three fluorine atoms at R_1.

There are pharmacological differences between these groups, but they are not sufficiently impressive, as far as I can judge, to enable one to distinguish sufficiently constant and characteristic effects in each group to develop even a tentative theory of neuro-pharmacological action in terms of variations in the phenothiazine structure.

However, the three groups do appear to differ in their relative anti-adrenergic and anti-cholinergic actions. Whereas the aliphatic derivatives have a relatively marked anti-adrenergic effect and a weak anti-cholinergic one, the reverse is the case with the piperidines such as mepazine; weight for weight the piperazines' adrenergic blocking activity resemble chlorpromazine, but in clinical practice, because of the smaller dose required, autonomic effects are much less conspicuous. The three chemical groups also differ in their effects on the motor system. Both the aliphatic and piperazine group diminish psychomotor over-activity but the latter will often stimulate activity in inert patients. The piperazines are able to block conditioned avoidance responses more effectively. The anti-emetic effects of the piperazines are greater; as also is potentiation of the effects of other sedatives, such as barbiturates.

Of more theoretical interest is some recent work (admittedly on frogs) which suggests the groups act differentially on a hypophyseal suppressor area in the hypothalamus, with the release of the melanocyte stimulating hormone from the pituitary. Scott investigated 10 phenothiazines.[5] Those in the piperazine group with fluorine at R_1 stimulated the production of the hormone more than did the piperazines without fluorine. The other piperazines were more active in this respect than were the derivatives with the aliphatic group; but the piperidines were inactive.

The relative tranquillizing potencies of the derivatives[6] and their overall therapeutic effects are functions of greater practical interest: of equal importance are differences in their ability to relieve specific clinical symptoms, or to affect other characteristics of patients.

Two carefully designed studies, one at Spring Grove State Hospital[7] and the other in which many of the Veterans Administration Hospitals[8] collaborated, compared five and six different phenothiazines respectively in the treatment of schizophrenia. In both studies the representative of the piperidine group, mepazine, was less effective than were the other derivatives. Promazine, which has an aliphatic side-chain and no halogen, was the next least effective. Although the differences between the remainder were not significant the three piperazine derivatives more consistently ranked high than did the other groups. The acutely ill patients on the piperazine derivatives in the Spring Grove study became less withdrawn than did those on the aliphatic ones; the piperidine, mepazine, was least successful in lessening withdrawal. On the other hand the aliphatic derivative, chlorpromazine, was most effective in improving thought disorder.[9]

Many other clinical comparisons have been made between two or more phenothiazine derivatives. The consensus of these is that the piperazine derivatives are between 3 and 10 times as potent as are the aliphatic ones, and that when halogen atoms are substituted at position R_2 potency is increased also. The piperazines also appear to be more effective with apathetic withdrawn patients, while the restless and agitated benefit from the aliphatic group.

Marks attempted to predict the individual's response to phenothiazine derivatives by relating their response scores to their initial ratings on a number of measures of behaviour.[10] Responsiveness to chlorpromazine was associated with co-operativeness; response to the piperazine, trifluoperazine, with anxiety and tension, and the other piperazines with sociability and with activity. Although this study used a fresh approach to the problem of the relations between the phenothiazine derivatives and patients' behaviour the findings again leave one uncertain about the clinical (and pharmacological) significance of the associations found so far.

The type and incidence of side effects and of toxic effects are modified by the nature of the substitutions both in position R_2 and in position R_1. Autonomic side effects occur most frequently with the aliphatic group, as does drowsiness, but extrapyramidal symptoms are much more common with the piperazine derivatives, especially those in which CF_3 is substituted. Forced restlessness is another syndrome which is more likely to occur with the piperazine side-chain. Toxic effects on the liver, however, are relatively infrequent in this group. The piperidine side-chain is associated more with parasympathetic side effects.

DiMascio, Havens and Klerman studied the relations between the chemical structure of the phenothiazines and their actions on selected physiological and performance functions in normal males.[11, 12] The two aliphatic phenothiazines, at peak time of action, produced confusion, impaired psychomotor performance, causing inco-ordination and a decrease in tapping speed, and performance on cognitive tests; the autonomic effects found were a fall of blood pressure and constriction of the pupil. The piperazines by contrast, produced no or very few effects of this kind; rather they improved performance on motor tests and cognitive tasks. The authors, however, could find no key behavioural or pharmacologic effect which was characteristic of all the therapeutically active phenothiazines, and which distinguished the clinically effective from ineffective derivatives.

This conclusion summarizes one of the main problems: although the phenothiazine derivatives have some distinctive pharmacological and psychological effects, their therapeutic efficacy does not relate consistently to these. The chemical structural features of the phenothiazines, therefore, have not so far been found to have a sufficiently constant association with pharmacological, psychological *and* clinical effects to develop a theory of their mode of action and provide direction to research.

I would like to end by suggesting a way in which *clinical* research might contribute to differentiating the specific effects of the phenothiazine derivatives and the clinical indications for their use. This could be done by using an extended cross-over design in which each patient is given two different phenothiazines on *two* or more occasions. By alternating the two treatments at least twice, those patients could be identified who respond consistently to one of the treatments and not to the other. Their different clinical and psychological characteristics, as well as any differences in pharmacological effects on them could then be compared and analysed.

REFERENCES

1. HIMWICH, H. E., RINALDI, F. and WILLIS, D. J., *J. nerv. ment. Dis.* **124**, 53 (1956).
2. LEWIS, J. J., *Introduction to Pharmacology*, 2nd ed., p. 221. Livingstone, London, (1962).
3. WERNER, G., *Amer. J. med. Sci.* **237**, 631 (1959).
4. BRADLEY, P. B., In *Physiological Pharmacology*, I, Eds. Root, W. S. and Hoffman, F. G Academic Press, London (1962).
5. SCOTT, G. T., *Psychopharm. Serv. Centre Bull.* **2**, 58 (1962).
6. AYD, F. J., *J. med. Soc. N.J.* **57**, 4 (1960).
7. KURLAND, A. A., HANLON, T. E., TATOM, M. H., OTA, K. Y. and SIMOPOULOS, A. M., *J. nerv. ment. Dis.* **133**, 1 (1961).
8. CASEY, J. F., LASKY, J. J., KLETT, C. J. and HOLLISTER, L. E., *Amer. J. Psychiat.* **117**, 97 (1960).
9. KURLAND, A. A., MICHAUX, M. H., HANLON, T. E., OTA, K. Y. and SIMOPOULOS, A. M., *J. nerv. ment. Dis.* **134**, 48 (1962).
10. MARKS, J., *J. nerv. ment. Dis.* **137**, 597 (1963).
11. DIMASCIO, A., HAVENS, L. L. and KLERMAN, G. L., *J. nerv. ment. Dis.* **136**, 15 (1963).
12. DIMASCIO, A., HAVENS, L. L. and KLERMAN, G. L., *J. nerv. ment. Dis.* **136**, 168 (1963).

USE OF OTHER DRUGS
IN THE TREATMENT OF THE SCHIZOPHRENIC

W. H. Trethowan

Summary—The treatment of schizophrenia by non-phenothiazine drugs does not yet seem to produce measurable advantages over those which can be obtained with phenothiazines either alone or in some cases in combination with other agents. However, if no better than phenothiazines, some may produce comparable effects. At present, those most worthy of further study appear to be the butyrophenones and possibly oxypertine also.

Résumé—Le traitement de la schizophrénie par les médicaments non phénothiaziniques ne semble pas présenter des avantages mesurables sur ceux offerts par les phénothiazines administrées soit seules, soit dans quelques cas, en association avec d'autres agents. Cependant, s'ils ne sont pas supérieurs aux phénothiazines, certains peuvent produire des effets comparables. A l'heure actuelle, ce sont les butyrophénones et peut-être l'oxpertine aussi qui semblent justifier le plus d'amples recherches.

Zusammenfassung—Die Behandlung der Schizophrenie mit Medikamenten, die nicht der Phenothiazinreihe angehören, scheint bis jetzt keine erfassbaren Vorteile gegenüber der Therapie mit Phenothiazinen allein oder in Verbindung mit anderen Substanzen zu bieten. Immerhin zeitigen einige Präparate zwar nicht bessere Ergebnisse als die Phenothiazine, aber doch vergleichbare. Gegenwärtig scheinen die Butyrophenone und möglicherweise auch Oxpertin diejenigen zu sein, die weitere Erforschung am meisten rechtfertigen.

UNTIL the identification of schizophrenia and its separation from the amorphous aggregate of insanity no rational treatment was possible. The luckless victim was subjected, regardless of his needs and in common with a multitude of sufferers from other unidentified mental disorders to bleeding, clysters, blisters, tartar emetic, croton oil and other primitive forms of shock treatment. Later, as chemical began to replace mechanical means of restraint, the more inconvenient behaviour of schizophrenics was often suppressed under an umbrella of chronic bromide intoxication.

Even in more recent times the drug treatment of schizophrenia can be likened to a retreat from a battlefield along a road on which numerous casualties are strewn. While these casualties consist mostly of other ranks and " also rans ", they include at least one field marshal—insulin!

Following the advent of the phenothiazines and certain other drugs which have been shown to have more definite effects upon schizophrenic symptoms the battle has not gone quite so unremittingly in favour of the enemy. But it is far from won and while we proceed along largely empirical lines, further casualties must inevitably occur.

There is a lesson to be learned from this. Although we are now able to identify schizophrenia with some degree of accuracy and some current concepts of its nature appear to possess validity there is still much inexactitude. This is all too apparent in scanning the now vast literature concerning the effects of a host of drugs upon the symptoms of schizophrenia, if not on the disorder itself. As a recent writer has stated:[1] " There is room for more reports involving the application of skill, experience and judgement to clinical work and observation, to supplement the many bald statistical reports of miscellaneous populations labelled schizophrenic or neurotic ".

My brief is to review the treatment of schizophrenia by other drugs; that is by drugs other than phenothiazines, which still have pride of place.

An attempt to classify these drugs suggests that they fall into two main types. In the first category are those largely used as adjuvants, either to deal with symptoms which phenothiazines or ECT do not readily control or, as in the case of anti-parkinsonian agents, to subdue side effects. Also included in this category are various endocrine preparations such as anabolic steroids, dehydroisoandrosterone, oestrogen or stilboestrol, or substances such as norethandrolone which may help to control pre-menstrual tension which in some female schizophrenic patients may lead to a periodic exacerbation of symptoms.[2]

Another subgroup consists of drugs which may be roughly classified as psychoenergizers, by reason of their producing increased activity, heightening mood or overcoming anergia (itself either an intrinsic part of some schizophrenic syndromes or an outcome of treatment with phenothiazines). Or yet again, drugs which unlike phenothiazines appear to act on the higher rather than the lower brain centres and which may play a limited and usually only a secondary part in controlling anxiety or agitation: drugs such as meprobamate, propanedial dicarbamate, diazepam, chlordiazepoxide, none of which appear to be any more effective in schizophrenia than that old standby amylobarbitone.

The second broad category contains drugs which differ in chemical structure from the phenothiazines but produce very similar psychotropic or neuroleptic effects and in some cases very similar side effects, in particular extrapyramidal symptoms. These include reserpine, tetrabenazine and benzquinamide which are chemically closely related and resemble reserpine; oxypertine, a psychotropic drug containing an indole ring and related to tryptophan; and the butyrophenones of which several types are now in fairly wide use.

Of the various endocrine preparations used in the hope of controlling schizophrenia, thyroid seems to have been one of the first to receive the death knell. If the use of thyroid ever had any rational basis, this must have been the outcome of a hope that it would stimulate withdrawn and apathetic schizophrenics into activity, perhaps by raising their basal metabolic rate. Alternatively its use may have seemed justified to some on account of Gjessing's discovery that the administration of thyroxine resolved periodic catatonia by restoring a normal nitrogen balance. Whatever the basis of this therapy, schizophrenics were at one time prescribed thyroid sometimes in enormous quantities. Luckily and possibly by reason of the peculiar non-responsiveness of schizophrenics to various hormones including thyroid[3] the treatment, if it did no good seems to have done little harm.

Insulin is worthy of a better epitaph. Although it is now clear that insulin coma had no specific effect there can be little doubt that some schizophrenics obtained benefit from this treatment, at least for a time. This seems to have been the outcome, possibly, of three factors. First, insulin coma therapy sometimes greatly improved the physical health of debilitated schizophrenic patients. Many put on weight and *pari passu* with improved physical well-being, some resolution of anxiety and tension occurred. Secondly, many of the doctors and nurses responsible for carrying out this onerous procedure, one by no means without risk, not only had considerable faith in the outcome of treatment—perhaps more so in the earlier rather than in the later stages—but became more than ordinarily interested in the welfare of those under-going the treatment. Not for nothing perhaps was the statement once made that a sure way to boost the morale of a mental hospital was to start an insulin coma unit. The third and related factor seems to have been that an insulin unit facilitated the creation of a then peculiar group situation from which some patients at least derived therapeutic benefit and which was not easy to reproduce by any other means.

Of other endocrine treatments it was inevitable that corticotrophin and cortisone should have been tried. While initial reports were encouraging properly controlled studies using a relatively high dosage over a prolonged period gave unequivocally negative results.[4] In view of the psychotogenic effects of high dosage steroids in some patients[5] matters might have been made worse. But this, again perhaps due to the general or biological non-responsiveness of schizophrenics, seems not to have occurred.

In 1952, Strauss *et al.*[6] gave preliminary encouraging reports of the use of dehydroisoandrosterone. The drug was said to have euphoriant properties and to increase self-confidence in those constitutionally immature schizo-phrenics exhibiting prolonged pubertal crises rather than true process schizophrenia. In a subsequent paper Sands[7] stated that although dehy-droisoandrosterone " is not a treatment for schizophrenia . . . and indeed may make some patients worse, its use at a certain stage and in conjunction with other methods may be useful ". Following this, dehydroisoandrosterone seems to have fallen largely into disuse.

The latest fashion in endocrine treatment appears to be for anabolic steroids. Some initial reports of the use of oxymetholone though only as an adjunct were encouraging. Of 28 hospitalized schizophrenics reported by Lapinsohn[8] all improved, in 22 cases the response being recorded as excellent or good; in the remaining 6, fair. The response of 15 schizophrenic outpatients was less striking though it was said that only one failed to improve.

Barron, Rudy and Smith[9] who compared carphenazine with oxymetholone were less enthusiastic. Although they felt that the euphoriant action of oxymetholone was useful as an adjunctive treatment in schizophrenia they recorded increase in agitation in some cases and expressed doubt in identifying those patients who who could be expected to respond best.

More recently Tarlo, Zachariadis and Marks[10] found no change in 10 chronic schizophrenics following the administration of anabolic steroids apart from one patient who apparently improved spontaneously 6 months after completion of the trial. It looks, therefore, as if anabolic steroids like diandrone may also find a place on the casualty list.

Of potentially greater interest is the use of oestrogens or stilboestrol for the control of sexual symptoms in male schizophrenics. If repressed homosexuality really plays a part in the genesis of paranoid reactions in males as Freud[11] postulated, the suppression of sexuality by oestrogens or stilboestrol might be expected, on theoretical grounds at least, to cause some benefit to those in this category. As is well known, stilboestrol judiciously used to suppress libido will sometimes keep selected sexual offenders out of trouble.

In practice, however, the administration of oestrogens or stilboestrol appears to have no effect on the course of a schizophrenic illness other than the adjunctive effect of suppressing sexual preoccupation or inconvenient sexual behaviour such as overt masturbation in some but not all patients [12] Those patients who improve in this way also seem to gain weight; in those who do not gain, improvement may only be temporary or deterioration may occur.

It appears then as if the effects of real or synthetic oestrogens on schizophrenic patients differ in no essential respect from that on other non-schizophrenics who have sexual problems, i.e. sexual drive is reduced in some cases, which may of course be convenient, but without amelioration of the underlying disorder. Anyway Freud's contention is arguable as a study carried out by Planasky and Johnston[13] of the incidence of heterosexual problems and homosexual concerns in 150 hospitalized male schizophrenics seems to show. They found no significant relationship between the degree of paranoidness exhibited and heterosexual or homosexual concerns in psychosis, the main conclusion being that paranoid development and homosexuality as found in schizophrenics are not specifically related to one another.

Various recommendations have been made for adjuvant drug therapy of other types including vitamins. Hoffer[14] in a double-blind trial found that schizophrenics responded more satisfactorily and remained better after discharge if nicotinic acid (or nicotinamide) in daily doses of 3 g was included in treatment for periods of at least 30 days. Milner[15] also found that some chronic psychiatric patients, mainly those with affective symptoms but some with paranoid symptom-complexes also, received benefit from saturation with ascorbic acid. Although treatment with vitamins seems almost to savour of a bygone age both these are fairly recent papers.

A number of drugs, other than those such as orphenadrine given specifically to counter anti-parkinsonian effects, have been or are being used in conjunction with phenothiazines. The results seem somewhat variable. Using combinations of chlorpromazine with other drugs, viz. dexamphetamine, isocarboxazid, trifluoperazine and imipramine in chronic schizophrenia Casey et al.[16] found none of these combinations superior to chlorpromazine alone. In the case of dexamphetamine matters were made worse as this increased hostility, paranoid belligerency and thought disorder. Indeed as a general rule the amphetamines are strongly contra-indicated in schizophrenia.

On the whole, combinations of phenothiazines, with antidepressive drugs are not widely reported. Perhaps, however, they are more favoured than written about. Cheng and Fogel[17] used a combination of trifluoperazine and amitriptyline in the treatment of 100 women with paranoid schizophrenia and claimed considerable improvement in 73. A similar improvement was also noted in 25 other female patients suffering from a paranoid psychosis not connected with schizophrenia. Owing to the affective component often evident in schizophrenic as well as non-schizophrenic paranoid states, there may be some rational basis for a combination of neuroleptic and antidepressive medication using imipramine or amitriptyline though, with some possible exceptions,[18] not monoamine oxidase inhibitors which like amphetamine are generally contra-indicated. Amitriptyline which is also said to counter some of the cataleptic effects of phenothiazines may also be used to counteract the depression which long-continued administration of these drugs produces in certain schizophrenic patients.

Some other drugs have been used to counteract the inactivity which chronic schizophrenics exhibit and which may be augmented by neuroleptic drugs. Acetoxymethane hydrochloride has been said to have such a psychotonic effect.[19] In animal experiments the drug diminishes the side effects of phenothiazines and counteracts their cataleptic action. In humans while it has been regarded as a useful supportive drug therapy during neuroleptic treatment in that it makes patients more active, there is thought to be some risk of habituation.[20] As there seem to be no very recent reports of its use it may have proved less effective than first thought or some disadvantage may have been uncovered.

G

We may now turn and consider the treatment of schizophrenia by other non-phenothiazine neuroleptics. Reserpine which came into use about 1953, not long after chlorpromazine first appeared, has now largely fallen out of fashion. While reserpine and other rauwolfia alkaloids are psychotropic and exert a favourable action on some schizophrenic syndromes[21] there seems to be general agreement that the drugs are less effective than phenothiazines,[22] that their action is much slower[23] and that in some cases, at least, side effects are more troublesome, in particular the tendency of rauwolfia alkaloids to produce depression, especially in those with a schizo-affective type of psychosis.[24]

Two synthetics tetrabenazine and benzquinamide which act similarly to reserpine have aroused some favourable comments.[25, 26] In one study the results suggested that benzquinamide in doses of up to 1200 mg daily was effective in many newly admitted schizophrenics.[25] The drug was said to have the greatest effect on emotional withdrawal, conceptual disorganization, tension, suspiciousness, hallucinations, unusual thought content and blunted affect. Although these agents have the advantage over reserpine of speedier action, side effects are frequent and may be troublesome. Weakness, fatigue, drowsiness, anxiety, agitation and in some cases, excitement occur; also extrapyramidal symptoms including dystonic reactions.

Another double-blind comparison of benzquinamide with chlorpromazine, and a placebo was less favourable.[27] Once again, extreme agitation and a general exacerbation of psychotic symptoms including depression were observed in some patients receiving benzquinamide and the final results of treatment with this drug were less beneficial than those obtained with chlorpromazine. It was stated that 800 mg was the maximum safe daily dosage and, like reserpine, that the drug should be used with great caution in patients suffering from schizophrenia with a depressive component.

A number of recent papers have commented favourably on oxypertine.[28] Calwell, Jacobsen and Skarbek[29] compared it with trifluoperazine in the treatment of chronic schizophrenic females, and concluded that oxypertine may be superior especially in its effect on certain types of psychotic behaviour and in increasing the ability of the patients to communicate. Side effects so far recorded have included vomiting, giddiness, transient photophobia, and parkinsonian symptoms. Varying degrees of motor restlessness, occasionally accompanied by anxiety and panic, may occur at a dosage of 120–160 mg daily but subside within 2 or 3 days of withdrawal. While the drug does not appear to be overtly hepatotoxic, abnormally high transaminase values and a raised alkaline phosphatase have been found in a number of patients.

Last but not least consideration will be given to the butyrophenones. Some 4000 different drugs of this class have been synthesized by Janssen in Belgium, but only a few have been tried out on human subjects. In this country haloperidol is the only one so far to have received much attention, though in Birmingham we have recently concluded a pilot trial of tri-fluoperidol on chronic schizophrenic patients.

Haloperidol can be considered as a prototype of this class of drugs. Its pharmacological action bears a general resemblance to that of the phenothiazines but is reputed to be more specific and to have a greater degree of penetration. It has powerful neuroleptic and psychotropic effects and within the therapeutic dose range is said to be free of autonomic and idiosyncratic side effects. Thus orthostatic hypotension, sympathicomimetic effects and a variety of sensitivity reactions familiar in the case of phenothiazines are said not to occur. What haloperidol and other butyrophenones do strongly tend to produce are extrapyramidal symptoms including rigidity, tremor, akathisia, torsion spasm, etc., which in the event of over-dosage can be severe.

Although fairly good results have been claimed in the treatment of affective disorders by haloperidol, in particular manic states, its superiority to phenothiazines in schizophrenia is not yet fully established. In one study haloperidol was found to be slightly better than a placebo though its superiority to previous medication did not reach statistical significance.[30] In another its antipsychotic action and overall clinical efficacy were found to be on a par with those of chlorpromazine though it was suggested that the two drugs achieved their effects in different ways.[31]

Reports from Europe have, on the whole, been more favourable though it should be noted that many continental psychiatrists do not favour the double-blind controlled type of trial customary in the United Kingdom. In any event the tendency of butyrophenone drugs to produce extrapyramidal symptoms at a relatively low dosage level makes a blind trial difficult although not impossible as these effects can be minimized by anti-parkinsonian drugs which can be given in conjunction with a placebo as well.

Some German psychiatrists believe that the psychotropic and extrapyramidal effects of the drug are related and that the maximum psychotropic effect is achieved just at that point where minimal extrapyramidal signs occur. Several tests may be employed to assess this, the simplest using handwriting. In practice haloperidol or trifluoperidol are administered in increasing doses and the subjects requested to copy a four-line poem daily. The first sign of extrapyramidal disturbance is revealed by cramping of the lettering, shortening of the lines and increased illegibility. While other more refined techniques can be employed, e.g. tracing a pencil line in a maze or measuring the regularity of sustained pressure on an ergograph these seem to be more elaborate procedures having little advantage over handwriting tests. Although extrapyramidal symptoms can fairly readily be controlled there is thought to be no advantage to be gained from increasing the dosage to the point where grosser extrapyramidal symptoms occur as these may detract from the overall therapeutic efficacy of the drugs.

Depending on the level of dosage employed, three general kinds of response to haloperidol are said to occur. The first which occurs at minimum dosage is a general tranquillizing or slightly sedative effect. In larger doses haloperidol may have a stimulating effect which is said to activate anergic patients, break up autistic patterns of behaviour and enhance co-operation in psychological and work therapies. This range of effect extends, in terms of dosage, up to the point where neuroleptic signs occur as indicated by the appearance of slight extrapyramidal signs. Within this range haloperidol has a psychotropic action leading to the abolition of agitation, aggressive behaviour and motor restlessness. This may be accompanied by diminished preoccupation with secondary psychotic symptoms, e.g. delusions and hallucinations though how much these kinds of symptoms are ameliorated seems to depend to some extent on the chronicity of the condition. The actual dose required in any individual must be determined by trial and error. This again makes a double-blind trial difficult. Roughly the equipotency of haloperidol in terms of its neuroleptic effect in a dosage range of 2·5–8·5 mg/70 kg body weight daily, can be compared to that of trifluoperazine in a daily dosage range of 15–30 mg.

As already stated opinions vary as to the effect of haloperidol on schizophrenia. While some maintain that the best results occur in acute cases it is admitted that these often respond equally satisfactorily to phenothiazines. Others believe that it is in chronic schizophrenia that haloperidol is most effective, leading to a reduction in autism, improvement in interpersonal relationships and increased co-operation in treatment programmes. Secondary symptoms such as delusions may not respond though it is said that these can be " broken up " by the judicious use of ECT with which haloperidol may be combined. The best response is recorded in paranoid and catatonic states but, as with other forms of treatment, hebephrenics appear to respond less well.

Trifluoperidol has psychopharmacological effects closely resembling those of haloperidol but is more powerful. The relationship between these two drugs appears to be somewhat analogous to that between chlorpromazine and trifluoperazine. Neuroleptic effects with trifluoperidol can occur within a daily dosage range as low as 1·0–1·5 mg. As in the case of haloperidol autonomic effects are absent at this dosage level though it is said to differ from haloperidol inasmuch that at very low dosage little or no tranquillizing effect is seen but a greater stimulating effect which can excite agitated patients to their disadvantage. While the main indications resemble those for haloperidol, trifluoperidol is said to give the greatest benefit in acute and subacute schizophrenic states. While it may produce aggression in some autistic patients this is thought to be prognostically favourable.

We have recently concluded a pilot study in Birmingham of the effect of trifluoperidol on 37 chronic schizophrenic patients (16 males, 21 females).

The study was carried out independently by 6 different consultants in 5 hospitals according to a pre-arranged plan and no notes were compared until after the trial was concluded. The patients were very much " hard core cases " the length of continuous stay in hospital varying from 1 to 41 years (mean 17·5 years). All patients showed considerable personality deterioration, social withdrawal, apathy and anergia. Attempts at occupational therapy and social rehabilitation had been largely unsuccessful despite extensive use of the whole range of ataractic drugs.

As a whole the therapeutic results were unimpressive, though it must always be borne in mind that these were particularly chronic patients unlikely to respond to any kind of treatment. Some evidence of definite clinical improvement occurred in 4 instances. In 9 others a slight improvement was seen. Of the remainder 20 showed no change and 4 were slightly worse. Eight out of 19 patients who developed some extrapyramidal signs showed some improvement compared with 5 of the 18 in whom no extrapyramidal signs occurred. This difference is small and insufficient to substantiate the hypothesis that neuroleptic and psychotropic effects are associated.

Of the patients who definitely improved all 4 were male but the clinical features they showed did not serve to differentiate them from the remainder of the group. The improvement occurred early, within 2 weeks and was maintained on a dose of 4 mg daily. In all cases a sharp deterioration was noted 7 days after withdrawal of the drug. What we did discover was that these patients tolerated a much higher dosage than that advocated by continental investigators. For example on doses as high as 10·5 mg daily only 19 patients developed parkinsonian signs the critical dosage for this development lying between 2·75 and 7·75 mg daily.

Dr. R. H. Cawley, to whom I am grateful for allowing me to quote these results, concluded: " It appears that triperidol has a variable neuroleptic action and a variable psychotropic action in the sample of the chronic population studied. There is no association between these two effects. These conclusions apply only to relatively short-term administration of the drug, in the stated dosage, to the present sample of hospitalized chronic schizophrenic patients ".

It would appear however that chronic schizophrenics have a greater tolerance or resistance to trifluoperidol as opposed to recent and more acute cases in whom the clinical response is said to be better but who develop extrapyramidal signs at a much lower dosage. However, good results in chronic schizophrenia have been claimed in at least one American study[32] in which trifluoperidol was compared with chlorpromazine in chronic schizophrenics who had received no medication for 60 days prior to the start of the trial. The investigators concluded that during 4 years of double-blind studies trifluoperidol was the only experimental drug that surpassed chlorpromazine in therapeutic efficacy. The drug therefore appears to be worthy of further appraisal, in particular the claim that it has been used successfully in autistic children.

Of the other butyrophenones fairly extensive trials have been carried out of dipiperon. Its effects seem to place it in a somewhat different class. Firstly, it has fewer neurological effects and where parkinsonian symptoms do occur these tend to be transient. In contrast the drug has a more powerful sedative effect and a much greater autonomic effect. Thus it bears a closer resemblance to chlorpromazine than does haloperidol or trifluoperidol. Clinically it is reported to have, in addition, a special effect on mood, what the continental psychiatrists term a " mood-harmonizing " effect. It is said to increase affective responses in patients who are autistic and to elevate mood in schizophrenic patients who are depressed, though having little effect where depression is the primary diagnosis. It may have some indications therefore in schizo-affective states and in some types of paranoid schizophrenia. It is difficult to obtain a definite opinion as to its value. One fairly recent report while showing improvement in some cases gave fairly equivocal results. Side effects, in particular hypotension seem to have been troublesome.[33]

Yet another butyrophenone, haloanisone compares to prochlorperazine in its effects, these being sedative, autonomic and neuroleptic. It is thought to be useful in veterinary medicine as it reduces cannibalistic tendencies in animals such as occur in a disorder affecting pigs which apparently causes them to chew one another's tails. Its application to the control of psychiatric disorders in man is uncertain. While it is said to be one of the fastest acting of all neuroleptics and therefore might have some use in the control of acute delirious states, in other respects it can be described as a straight-forward chlorpromazine competitor. A fairly recent study suggested a favourable effect on 20 of 35 patients suffering from a mixed bag of psychiatric disorders. Side effects of various kinds occurred in approximately one-quarter of the cases.[34] There are other reports that it is poorly tolerated.[1]

REFERENCES

1. WORTIS, J., *Amer. J. Psychiat.* **120**, 643 (1964).
2. SWANSON, D. W., BARRON, A., FLOREN, A. and SMITH, J. A., *Amer. J. Psychiat.* **120**, 1101 (1964).
3. HOSKINS, R. G., *Biology of Schizophrenia*, Norton, New York, 1946.
4. REES, L. and KING, G. M., *J. ment. Sci.* **102**, 155 (1956).
5. TRETHOWAN, W. H., *Acta psychiat. scand.* **29**, 243 (1954).
6. STRAUS, E. B., SANDS, D. E., ROBINSON, A. M., TINDALL, W. J. and STEVENSON, W. A. H., *Brit. med. J.* ii, 64 (1952).
7. SANDS, D. E., *J. ment. Sci.* **100**, 211 (1954).
8. LAPINSOHN, L. I., *Dis. nerv. Syst.* **23**, 226 (1962).
9. BARRON, A., RUDY, L. H. and SMITH, J. A., *Amer. J. Psychiat.* **119**, 1172 (1963).
10. TARLO, L., ZACHARIADIS, N. and MARKS, V., *Brit. J. Psychiat.* **110**, 287 (1964).
11. FREUD, S., *Introductory Lectures on Psycho-Analysis*, Allen and Unwin, London, 1922.

12. ADAMSON, J. D., *J. ment. Sci.* **105**, 762 (1959).
13. PLANANSKY, K. and JOHNSTON, R., *J. ment. Sci.* **108**, 604 (1962).
14. HOFFER, A., *Amer. J. Psychiat.* **120**, 171 (1963).
15. MILNER, G., *Brit. J. Psychiat.* **109**, 294 (1963).
16. CASEY, J. F., HOLLISTER, L. E., KLETT, C. J., LASKY, J. J. and CAFFEY, E. M., *Amer. J. Psychiat.* **117**, 997 (1961).
17. CHENG, S. F. and FOGEL, E. J., *Amer. J. Psychiat.* **119**, 780 (1963).
18. SAUNDERS, J. C., *Ann. N.Y. Acad. Sci.* **107**, 1081 (1963).
19. BAN, T. A. and ST. LAURENT, J., *J. Neuropsychiat.* **3**, 91 (1961).
20. BELLANDER–LOFVENBER, S., OSTERMAN, E. and BRATTEMO, C. E., *Nord. psykiat. T.* **15**, 141 (1961).
21. BOWER, H. M., *Med. J. Aust.* **1**, 268 (1957).
22. BLAIR, D., *Modern Drugs for the Treatment of Mental Illness*, Staples Press, London (1963).
23. PARE, C. M. B., *A Practical Introduction to Psychiatry*, Churchill, London (1964).
24. MOORE, J. N. P. and MARTIN, E. A., *Brit. med. J.* **1**, 8 (1957).
25. OVERALL, J. E., HOLLISTER, L. E., PARRETT, J. L., SHELTON, J. and CAFFEY, E. M., *Curr. ther. Res.* **5**, 335 (1963).
26. REES, L., *Postgrad. med. J.* **39**, 48 (1963).
27. BISHOP, M. P., GALLANT, D. M. and STEELE, C. A., *Curr. ther. Res.* **5**, 238 (1963).
28. DURELL, J. and POLLIN, W., *Brit. J. Psychiat.* **109**, 687 (1963).
29. CALWELL, W. P. K., JACOBSEN, M. and SKARBEK. *Brit. J. Psychiat.* **110**, 520 (1964).
30. OKASHA, A. and TEWFIK, G. I., *Brit. J. Psychiat.* **110**, 56 (1964).
31. HAWARD, L. R. C., *Brit. J. Psychiat.* **110**, 514 (1964).
32. GALLANT, D. M., BISHOP, M. P., TIMMONS, E. and STEELE, C. A., *Curr. ther. Res.* **5** 463 (1963).
33. NUYTS, A., *Acta neurol. belg.* **63**, 326 (1963).
34. KATILA, O. and PIIHKANEN, T., *Acta neurol. belg.* **63**, 291 (1963).

DISCUSSION

Opener: J. R. Smythies:

While the present symposium is primarily concerned with the present position of drugs used in psychiatry, it is important to look to the future too. I have, therefore, been asked to open this discussion by considering possible trends in the foreseeable future based on current research trends.

I think it is true to say that all the original members of the present drugs in use were discovered by an empirical process; that is by the astute utilization of some incidental observation and not by a systematic process of hypothesis, deduction and test. The use of the phenothiazines derived from the observation that a compound meant to be an anti-histamine had tranquillizing properties. The use of the MAOI's derived from the observation that an anti-tuberculous drug caused mood elevation and the imipramine group derived from a compound meant to be a tranquillizer. These drugs have proven successful and no doubt other drugs useful in psychiatry may be discovered in future in a similar manner: in such a case, of course, no predictions can be made.

It is, however, possible that treatments may be devised on a basis of our knowledge of aetiology—which is the rarely obtained ideal in medicine. Do we then have any notion of the possible aetiology, in biochemical terms, of the major diseases of psychiatry and, if so, do these notions suggest any therapy?

There are currently some working hypotheses in this field supported by a few slender strands of evidence. One growing point of psychiatric research today centres on the cerebral amines serotonin and noradrenaline and on the chemical process of methylation. There are three main planks on this platform.

The first is chemical. The major group of psychotomimetic drugs are N-methyl and/or O-methyl derivatives of serotonin, tryptamine or mescaline (Fig. 1). This surely must be of significance. For example (Fig. 1), bufotenin and psilocyn are the N.N. dimethyl derivatives of 5 HT and 4HT respectively and N.N. dimethyl tryptamine itself is a potent hallucinogen. Mescaline itself can be regarded as an O-methyl derivative of a catechol amine. Secondly, as Brune and Himwich[1] and Pollin et al.[2] have shown, the methyl donors methionine and betaine make schizophrenic symptoms worse in some cases.

Thirdly, Friedhoff and Van Winkle's[3] report that they have isolated the mescaline-like compound dimethoxyphenylethylamine (Fig. 2) from schizophrenic urine, offers support for this hypotheses as does Perry's[4] isolation of N-methyl adrenaline in excess amount from the urine of some schizophrenic children. Freidhoff's work has been confirmed by Clarke in this country[5] and by Sen and McGeer[6], Takasada et al.[7] and Kuehl et al.[8]

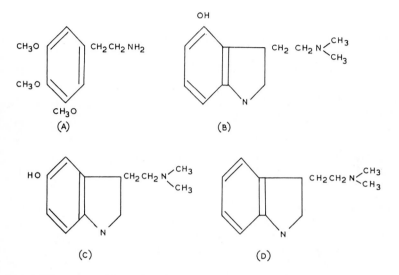

FIG. 1. The structural formulae of some hallucinogens (A) Mescaline (B) Psilocyn (C) Bufotenin (D) Dimethyl Tryptamine.

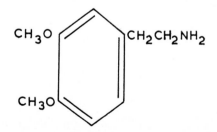

FIG. 2. Dimethoxyphenylethylamine—structural formula.

in North America and Japan. Perry et al.[9] were, however, unable to do so and they claim that this was the case because their patients had no fruit or vegetables in their diet for some days beforehand. However, as Freidhoff points out, they did not make their point by identifying dimethoxyphenylethylamine in the urine in any case *after* a diet containing fruit and vegetables. The matter is still, therefore, sub judice. It is, however, somewhat disappointing that five years after Seymour Kety's influential paper[10] stressing the absolute need for rigid dietary controls in this field that standards of dietary control are still so poor.

We can, however, make the tentative working hypothesis that disorders of serotonin or noradrenaline metabolism, particularly in the direction of excess methylation, may have something to do with psychoses. If this is the case, does the hypothesis suggest any possible lines of treatment? If the defect is one of excess methylation then feeding methyl acceptors might be useful. Hoffer et al.[11] have reported promising results from feeding large doses of nicotinamide but this has not been confirmed. Other methyl acceptors such as glycocyamine given alone are unfortunately too toxic for such use. Further work on these lines using some non-toxic methyl acceptor in graded doses would be useful. However, this does lead us to some suggestions for futher experiments to test the hypothesis. For example, we can ask: would methionine and betaine make schizophrenic symptoms worse if fed together with a methyl acceptor? Does feeding methionine or betaine increase the output of dimethoxyphenylethylamine in schizophrenia? Lastly one still urgently requires confirmation whether the excretion of this last compound is or is not an artefact of diet.

We can conclude that it is as yet too early to be able to do much in the way of deducing possible therapies from our knowledge of aetiology in this field, but at least we can see the way a little clearer as to what sort of experiments to do.

If we now consider the present remedies we can ask how does this model account for the action of current remedies—in particular the phenothiazines. It is possible that psychosis depends on two linked factors—an overactive central sympathetic system plus a metabolic fault in such a system. Most hallucinogenic drugs have effects on the central control of autonomic function—mostly sympatheticomimetic. One can imagine a metabolic fault that would not become manifest unless stress of a particular kind caused persistent over-activity of the central sympathetic system. This fault, once triggered, might lead to the internal production of hallucinogenic relatives of serotonin or catechol amines: hence more stress; thus a vicious circle would result. One way to break this circle would be to correct the metabolic fault. A method of doing this is not yet available to us. Another way may be to reduce the level of central sympathetic activity below " flash point ". This is how the phenothiazines may work.

Thus I would conclude that the present state of our knowledge of the biochemical concomitants of psychosis is not extensive enough to bear the weight of much speculation about possible therapy. Indeed, a great deal of work remains to be done in testing and developing the present hypotheses in this field—which it must be noted are still in an embryonic state. Indeed, some people would say that our knowledge of brain biochemistry is still so rudimentary that it is better to concentrate on building up this basic knowledge in the field of biological research in psychiatry rather than try and follow the will-of-the-wisp of speculative hypotheses. I would, however, argue that we need a balance between these two approaches and these hypotheses, sketchy as they are, deserve their share of development.

REFERENCES

1. Brune, G. C. and Himwich, H. E., *J. nerv. ment. Dis.* **134**, 447 (1962).
2. Pollin, W., Cardon, P. V. and Kety, S. S., *Science* **133**, 104 (1961).
3. Friedhoff, A. J. and Van Winkle, E., *J. nerv. ment. Dis.* **135**, 550 (1962).
4. Perry, T. L., *Science* **139**, 587 (1963).
5. Clarke, C. A., *Brit. med. J.* ii, 373 (1964).
6. Sen, N. P. and McGeer, P. L., *Biochem. biophys. Res. Commun.* **14**, 227 (1964).
7. Takesada, M., Kakimoto, Y., Sano, I. and Kaneko, Z., *Nature (Lond.)* **199**, 203 (1963).
8. Kuehl, F. A., Hichens, M., Ormond, R. E., Meisinger, M. A. P., Gale, P. H., Cirillo, V. J. and Brink, N. G., *Nature (Lond.)* **203**, 154 (1964).
9. Perry, T. L., Hansen, S. and McIntyre, L., *Nature (Lond.)* **202**, 519 (1964).
10. Kety, S. S., *Science* **129**, 1528 and 1590 (1959).
11. Hoffer, A., Osmond, H., Callbeck, M. J. and Kahan, I., *J. clin. exp. Psychopath.* **18**, 131 (1957).

Opener: K. Rawnsley:

Professor Trethowan likened the history of the treatment of schizophrenia to a retreat from a battlefield with many casualties by the wayside. In discussing insulin coma treatment he mentioned certain auxiliary factors which may have contributed to the therapeutic outcome, including the faith of doctors and nurses in the treatment, and a concentration of interest focussed upon the patient during the course. Also, he referred to the creation of a special group situation which would include both patients and staff.

I would like to follow this theme by considering certain aspects of environment, especially the social environment, which are relevant to the action of major tranquillizers.

Dr. Hordern and Professor Hamilton[1] drew attention in a paper last year to the importance of the institutional setting in which drugs are given. They quoted Faurbye[2] who pointed out that the most favourable reports of drug effectiveness have come from the mental hospitals which have the most meagre therapeutic resources.

Thus neuroleptic drugs have been acclaimed as miracle workers by the staffs of the vast State hospitals in the U.S.A. and of similar hospitals in other countries. Reports from small well-staffed psychotherapeutically oriented hospitals in the U.S. and from many hospitals in the U.K. have been more qualified and restrained.

There may, of course, be a number of possible explanations for these apparent differences in potency of the drugs. Variations in dosage or in attitudes of doctors may play a part. A clue to what I imagine could be the most plausible explanation is to be found in a study by Rathod[3] in which a programme of social activity in the ward was substituted for chlorpromazine therapy without any reversal of the improvement evidently brought about by the drug in the first place. Most of the patients were chronic schizophrenics. A sophisticated experiment to compare the effect of major tranquillizers with each other and with intensive social and nursing therapy has been reported by Professor Hamilton and his colleagues.[4] It was found that symptomatic improvement in chronic schizophrenics was produced equally, in males at any rate, by drugs as by social therapy. The two kinds of treatment exhibited simultaneously were not additive in their effects. One may conclude tentatively from this that the administration of phenothiazines in circumstances where active social treatment is already being pursued would make no difference or only a marginal difference to the clinical state in chronic schizophrenia.

Most clinical trials of the major tranquillizers in schizophrenia have been conducted in hospital. There are many advantages: relative simplicity of administration; strict control of experimental conditions; continuous observation and assessment of progress by professional personnel. It is well to remember, however, the limitations of this approach in view of present-day trends in psychiatric care. I refer to the shift of emphasis from intra- to extra-mural treatment for schizophrenia and other serious chronic disorders.

It should not be assumed that findings based on a trial of drugs conducted in a ward of chronic patients will be applicable to those who are living out of hospital and out of contact with other patients receiving similar medication.

Pharmacologists are well aware of the differences to be found between the effects of drugs on experimental animals treated singly in isolation and the effects observed when the animals are treated together as a group. Theoretically, therefore, it would be very desirable to arrange clinical trials of drugs using schizophrenic patients who are being cared for out of hospital. The difficulties of pursuing such investigations rigorously are obvious enough.

There is evidence that the post-hospital progress of the schizophrenic patient depends in part upon certain factors in the social environment—e.g. the type of living group to which he returns; the attitude of his family; the intensity of emotional contact with other members of the household. Drawing an analogy with the action of phenothiazines in the ward situation it may be that, in the presence of a favourable post-hospital social milieu, tranquillizers have little more to offer by way of clinical benefit. On the other hand, they may have a beneficial action in circumstances where the social climate is adverse.

It would be important to have more information about this question because the administration of phenothiazines for very long periods—especially to patients outside hospital—for whom the value may be marginal is obviously best avoided in view of the possible toxic effects.

So much for the importance of external environmental influences on the action of tranquillizers. What about the milieu intérieur? This is something one rarely hears about as an experimentally controlled variable in assessing the action of drugs. I do not know how important it would be in the case of the phenothiazines. Dr. Richter told us about the absorption and distribution of these drugs, but did not mention their fate. I was interested to note that at a recent meeting of the European Society for the Study of Drug Toxicity, Professor M. D. Milne drew attention to a striking variation in the stimulating action of amphetamine depending on urinary pH. The rate of elimination of certain drugs from the body is evidently very sensitive to changes in urinary acidity or alkalinity. If this kind of factor is important in controlling the excretion or perhaps even the destruction of other psychotropic drugs, then it must be reckoned with and, if necessary, controlled in clinical trials.

Looking through the literature on the comparison of one drug of the phenothiazine group with another in clinical trials, I have been struck by the frequency with which these trials are conducted at only one dose level for each drug. While acknowledging Professor Hamilton's remarks on the problem of multiplying variables in drug trials, I consider that a more sensible comparison could be achieved if each drug could be given at two dose levels at least.

REFERENCES

1. HORDERN, A. and HAMILTON, M., *Brit. J. Psychiat.* **109**, 500 (1963).
2. FAURBYE, A., In *Psychopharmacology Frontiers*, p. 245, Ed. Kline, N. S., Little, Brown, Boston, 1959.
3. RATHOD, N. H., *Lancet* **i**, 611 (1958).
4. HAMILTON, M., HORDERN, A., WALDROP, F. N. and LOFFT, J., *Brit. J. Psychiat.* **109**, 510 (1963).

GENERAL DISCUSSION

HAROLD PALMER (*St. Albans*): I cannot agree with Dr. Denham's statement about the value of thiopropazate in Huntington's chorea. Extensive studies in our hospital in this condition have suggested that it is useless.

DEREK RICHTER: Professor Trethowan spoke of thyroid treatment as belonging to the past. While I am sure that this is true in general, I think there have been cases reported where an occasional schizophrenic who is not apparently myxodematous has responded to thyroxin. I wonder if others have any experience of that?

W. A. H. STEVENSON (*London*): I have had similar experience to Dr. Richter with thyroid in one or two schizophrenics. I very much enjoyed Professor Trethowan's paper but I cannot let him bury dehydroisoandrosterone in a psychopharmacological " mass grave ". Strauss, I think, intended dehydroisoandrosterone not as a specific treatment for schizophrenia but for patients with a schizoid personality. With regard to it doing harm, it flared up aggression in the aggressive ones but this passed off when we stopped the drug.

F. A. JENNER: I should like to add something to what Dr. Richter said about thyroxin. In the M.R.C. Unit at Birmingham we have made attempts to repeat the work of Gjessing[1]. A patient with a periodic psychosis whom we studied every day for over two years showed good evidence for an alternate day syndrome for over ten years. We were able to stop it for eight days with thyroxin. Unfortunately the man developed auricular fibrillation for a short period and the experiment could not be continued at that time, but will be repeated. I think, however, that Professor Trethowan was referring more to the usual forms of schizophrenia rather than these periodic cases.

M. F. A'BROOK (*Northampton*): This morning Dr. Himwich I believe stated that the phenothiazines exerted an antidepressant effect as witnessed by the change in the EEG pattern, and Dr. Sainsbury says that the reverse pattern occurred. Can Dr. Sainsbury please elucidate this?

Secondly, clinical experience with the phenothiazines, especially chlorpromazine, suggest that they have a depressing effect. Some people have postulated that it is the build up of monoamines that is interfered with. I wonder if anyone has any comments on this?

P. SAINSBURY: I am really not familiar with all the literature on EEG and the phenothiazines but the difference may be in part due to different species. Dr. Himwich's slide was based on high doses given to rabbits. This may have some bearing on the differences. I believe there is some evidence that some of these phenothiazines, particularly the piperazine group do improve ratings of mood more than does chlorpromazine.

DEREK RICHTER: In answer to that question about chlorpromazine and brain amines, it was found that chlorpromazine influences the excretion products of the brain biogenic amines and, therefore, it was concluded by a number that that is part of their effect. Further investigation by Pletscher and also by Himwich's group showed that in these experiments the temperature of the animals had been allowed to fall and if they maintained the temperature then there was no effect on the excretion products.

A. PLETSCHER: I should like to modify some of the statements that Dr. Richter has just made. I agree that chlorpromazine and also haloperidol do not influence the total amine content of the brain, i.e. there is no build up of amines. However, the compounds do appear to affect the uptake of free amines into the storage sites or their attachment to the adrenergic receptor. Thus, chlorpromazine pretreatment counteracts the increase of noradrenaline due to administration of ^{14}C-DOPA. The ^{14}C-DOPA-induced rise of ^{14}C-phenolcarboxylic acids (metabolies of catecholamines) in the brain is, however, enhanced by chlorpromazine. Furthermore, Carlsson and co-workers showed that chlorpromazine and haloperidol enhance the increase of O-methylated catechol amines in the brain, which occurs after administration of an MAO inhibitor. As the amines cannot be stored, they are exposed to the catabolic enzymes and thus the cerebral content of some metabolies (e.g. phenolcarboxylic acids, O-methylated amines) is increased.

This effect is still found when the animal's temperature is maintained at a normal level.

M. F. A'BROOK (*Northampton*): If there is central amine block and a tendency for phenothiazines to produce depression should we not avoid phenothiazines in purely depressive illness?

J. M. HINTON (*London*): In answer to the question about the use of the phenothiazines in depressive illness, I should like to quote a paper of mine of 5 years ago[2] in which perphenazine, one of the piperazine group of the phenothiazines was used on a group of outpatients who had anxiety and depressive symptoms. Perphenazine (8 mg/day) was compared with a barbiturate and placebo. Whereas amylobarbitone and perphenazine both helped anxiety, depression was alleviated to some extent by perphenazine but not by amylobarbitone. I have rechecked the data and can find nothing wrong with the experimental method. On the other hand I do not find support in the literature of phenothiazines helping depression. Perhaps it was the group of patients that I chose or the low dose of perphenazine.

BERNARD B. BRODIE: There may be a partial answer. As a rule the tertiary amines of the chlorpromazine type tend to lose their sedative effect as you remove an N-methyl group. The body does this very neatly in the liver. For example, amitriptyline is sedative but on removal of one methyl group a very potent antidepressant nortriptyline is obtained. Likewise desmethyl imipramine does not show the chlorpromazine-like sedative effect of imipramine but is a powerful antidepressant.

J. MARKS: Professor Pletscher has spoken of the phenothiazines as blocking amine uptake into storage sites. Is this process an active one involving energy utilization, and can this be correlated with their reduction of energy release as reported by Dr. Richter?

A. PLETSCHER: I cannot answer that question. In all the experiments, environmental temperature of 30° to 31° and the body temperature has been carefully controlled, thus hypothermia is not likely to be a factor. I cannot say, however, whether it is an active process or whether it is just an interference with passive diffusion.

S. BOCKNER (*London*): I should like to return to the important question of the clinical use of phenothiazines in depression. I think that most clinical psychiatrists feel that phenothiazines are useful, combined with an antidepressant in the agitated case.

P. TURNER (*London*): I note in the paper by Dr. Richter that large amounts of phenothiazines are required to produce biochemical changes. While some psychiatrists use chlorpromazine in large doses, we have developed some tests of central function, which demonstrate a dose response effect of 10 and 25 mg chlorpromazine in normal subjects compared with a placebo. It would seem then that we should be able to find biochemical changes associated with tissue levels equivalent to a dose as low as 10 and 25 mg.

P. H. ROGERS (*Northampton*): The comments of Professor Rawnsley rather worry me. I come from a hospital which has been substantially transformed by the use of the phenothiazines. I do not believe that social factors are the whole answer. I can think of a number of patients who have lived for some time in a ward in which the environment has been substantially similar, apart from varying degrees of therapeutic social pressures. Amongst these patients in this relatively static environment some may be found in whom there is a critical dose level of phenothiazine. The astute sister will notice deterioration in these patients when the dose is reduced below this level. Such experience suggests that it is not only the social environment but also the chemical environment that has a part to play.

The other point which I feel merits more attention is the variation between patients in their response to different members of the phenothiazine group. One man's meat is another man's poison amongst the phenothiazine drugs.

C. P. B. BROOK (*Brentwood*): Before Professor Rawnsley sounds the Last Post over the phenothiazines, I think it is worth while examining a recent paper from St. Louis, Missouri,[3] which appeared in the *Journal of the American Medical Association* very recently called " Home versus Hospital Care for Schizophrenics ". The schizophrenics in this study were divided into two groups, one which went into hospital where they were treated by any means available. The second group received intensive treatment while remaining at home. The home care group did better than the hospital group. So far so good, but the home group were divided further into two groups—one group received placebos the second group received phenothiazine. It was the phenothiazine group of the home care patients who did best of all.

J. SCOTT (*Birmingham*): I would also support Dr. Rogers' comments on phenothiazines as adjuvants to continuous treatment of the schizophrenic. I have taken wards who have been on continuous phenothiazine therapy for periods of up to three or four years and en bloc have stopped their therapy with complete relapse. I would not accept that the hospital must therefore be automatically classed as a backwater.

D. C. WATT (*Aylesbury*): I would like to speak also on this question that Professor Rawnsley has raised. Most of the papers which Professor Rawnsley referred to were published at a time when very extravagant claims were being made for phenothiazines. There were stories of hospitals being emptied by their use. In our hospital among others we could not confirm these extravagant claims for the general hospital situation. That other factors are important is shown by another American study in which the discharge rate was improved in the hospital not only in the patients treated with the drugs but also in those not on the phenothiazines. We did see good effects in individual patients.

I cannot accept Dr. Scott's evidence on omitting treatment unless an identical placebo was substituted. If not, change of interest on the part of the staff might explain the findings.

W. H. TRETHOWAN: I feel that it may have been a remark of mine which influenced Professor Rawnsley's statement. I wish to rise in his defence at this particular point. I am sure that more has been read into Professor Rawnsley's remarks than he actually said. The lesson which he expressed and which ties up with a remark by Dr. Smythies is that treatment must remain empirical until we have a better understanding of aetiology. While treatment is empirical, we cannot neglect the psychological circumstances under which it is given.

J. DENHAM: I must agree with Dr. Palmer that in my experience too, thiopropazate is useless in Huntington's chorea. This does not, however, accord with most of the published literature. I found greater relief by giving thioproperazine in slowly increasing dosage until a mild parkinsonian tremor appears. The choreiform movements in Huntington's chorea then disappear.

I do not think I made myself clear about the use of the phenothiazines as antidepressants. Certainly some phenothiazine compounds have in my experience increased depression. On the other hand others seem to act as antidepressants in certain cases. The French in particular claim that levomepromazine has an antidepressant action. I cannot believe that these differences are as simple as dropping the methyl group as Dr. Brodie suggests.

Time did not allow me to enter into the question of social factors in the usage of phenothiazines.

K. Rawnsley: Mr. Chairman, I am delighted that my somewhat provocative remarks have caused Dr. Rogers and others to spring to the defence of the phenothiazine drugs. I was not, of course, trying to belittle these substances. I was merely sounding a note of caution.

REFERENCES

1. Gjessing, R., *Archiv. Psychiat. Nervenkr.* **200**, 366 (1959).
2. Hinton, J. M., *J. ment. Sci.* **105**, 872 (1959).
3. Pasamanick, Scarpitti, F. R., Lefton, M., Dinitz, S., Wernent, J. J. and McPheeters, H., *J. Amer. med. Ass.* **187**, 177 (1964).

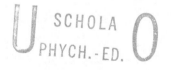

H

SESSION III
ANTIDEPRESSANTS
Chairman: Professor SIR AUBREY LEWIS

SOME CLINICAL ASPECTS OF ANTIDEPRESSANT DRUGS

C. M. B. PARE

Summary—Our own experience and that of other workers in the field support the view that the pharmacological separation of antidepressants into two distinct groups, the monoamine oxidase inhibitors and the imipramine group of drugs, holds true in clinical practice. Thus, if a patient fails to respond to a particular antidepressant after four weeks, he should be changed to a drug from the other group. The clinical impression that a patient failing to respond to an antidepressant after four weeks will be unlikely to improve more than partially if the drug is continued further, is supported as far as the monoamine oxidase inhibitors are concerned by the finding that 5-HT reaches a maximum in the human brain after four weeks administration.

There is fairly general agreement that the imipramine group of drugs should be tried first in the more endogenous types of depression, the monoamine oxidase inhibitors in the reactive and atypical cases, but more detailed descriptions of clinical indications for one or other group of antidepressants are subjects of controversy. This led to the suggestion that the response to a drug depended on the specific genetic type of the depression. Family studies support this thesis and work is continuing on these lines. It is accepted that the genetic factor is only one of many, influencing the response to antidepressant drugs. A biochemical aid would be invaluable to the clinician in his efforts to guess correctly which drug to use in any individual patient, but progress on these lines is fraught with difficulties.

In discussing side effects it was emphasized that these should be regarded as part of the normal action of the drug, are common to the group of drugs as a whole, and, at least with the monoamine oxidase inhibitors, are related to the potency of their antidepressant action. This was illustrated by some investigations using tryptophan where it was shown that just as this amino-acid increased the brain concentrations of active amines and relieved the patients' depression, so it increased total body amines and caused an increase in side effects. Toxic effects on the other hand are peculiar to the individual drug and not related to its antidepressant action. Although dramatic, toxic effects such as hepatic necrosis are rare and should be assessed in relation to the morbidity of the illness for which the drug may have to be prescribed.

Résumé—Notre propre expérience et celle d'autres auteurs dans ce domaine soutiennent le bien-fondé de la séparation pharmacologique des antidépressifs en deux groupes distincts, les inhibiteurs de la mono-amine oxydase et les substances du type de l'imipramine en pratique clinique. Donc si un malade ne répond pas à un agent antidépressif donné après quatre semaines, il faudra passer à une préparation de l'autre groupe. L'impression clinique qu'un malade n'ayant pas répondu au traitement par un antidépressif après quatre semaines sera vraisemblablement amélioré plus que partiellement, si on le poursuit, se trouve étayée, dans la mesure où, en ce qui concerne les inhibiteurs de la mono-amine oxydase, le 5-HT atteint un maximum dans le cerveau humain après une administration de quatre semaines.

Presque tous les auteurs sont d'accord sur le fait qu'il convient d'essayer d'abord les médicaments de la classe de l'imipramine dans les types de dépression plus endogènes et d'utiliser les inhibiteurs de la mono-amine oxydase dans les cas réactionnels et atypiques. Mais des descriptions plus détaillées des indications cliniques pour l'un ou l'autre groupe d'antidépressifs font l'objet de controverse. Ceci a suggéré que la réponse au traitement dépendait du type génétique spécifique de la dépression. Les études familiales viennent étayer cette thèse et des recherches sont poursuivies à ce sujet mais on admet que le facteur génétique est seulement un, parmi les nombreux facteurs, influençant la réponse de malade aux agents antidépressifs. Une aide biochimique serait inestimable pour le clinicien pour trouver exactement le médicament auquel il doit avoir recours dans le cas particulier, mais progresser dans cette voie se heurte à des difficultés.

En ce qui concerne les effets secondaires, on a souligné qu'ils doivent étre considérés comme faisant partie de l'action normale du médicament, qu'ils sont inhérents à ce groupe d'agents et en relation avec la puissance de leur effet antidépressif. Ceci a été illustré par quelques examens avec le tryptophane: de même que cet acide aminé accroît les concentrations des amines actives dans le cerveau et soulage la dépression, de même accroît-il les amines de l'organisme tout entier et provoque partant une augmentation des effets secondaires. D'autre part, les effets toxiques sont particuliers à la préparation donnée et ne sont pas liés à son action antidépressive. Bien que des réactions toxiques dramatiques telles que la nécrose hépatique soient rares, elles doivent être évaluées en fonction de la morbidité de la maladie pour laquelle la préparation a été prescrite.

Zusammenfassung—Unsere eigene Erfahrung und diejenige anderer Autoren, die sich mit diesem Gebiet befassen, bestätigen die Auffassung, dass sich die pharmakologische Unterteilung der Antidepressiva in Monoaminoxydase-Hemmer und Medikamente, die dem Imipramin verwandt sind, klinisch als richtig erweist. Der klinische Eindruck, bei einem Patienten, der innerhalb von 4 Wochen auf ein Antidepressivum nicht anspricht, sei kaum mehr als eine teilweise Besserung zu erwarten, wird für die MAO-Hemmer durch die Tatsache bestätigt, dass die Höchstkonzentration von 5-HT im menschlichen Hirn nach vierwöchiger Verabreichung erreicht wird.

Man ist sich allgemein darüber einig, dass die Imipramin-Analoga bei endogenen Depressionen zuerst verabreicht werden sollten, während bei reaktiven oder atypischen Formen eher den MAO-Hemmern der Vorzug zu geben ist; detailliertere Angaben über die klinischen Indikationen der einen oder der anderen Medikamenten-Gruppe sind indessen umstritten, was zu der Vermutung führte, das Ansprechen auf ein Medikament hänge von dem spezifischen genetischen Typ der Depression ab. Untersuchungen an Familien unterstützen diese Hypothese, deren Prüfung weiter verfolgt wird, man nimmt aber an, der genetische Faktor sei nur einer von vielen, die das Ansprechen auf ein Antidepressivum beeinflussen. Die Hilfe des Biochemikers wäre von unschätzbarem Wert für den Kliniker, der bemüht ist, richtig zu erraten, welches Präparat bei dem einzelnen Patienten zu geben wäre, aber ein Fortschritt in dieser Richtung ist mit vielen Schwierigkeiten verbunden.

Bei der Diskussion der Nebenwirkungen wurde betont, dass sie als ein Teil der eigentlichen Wirkung dieser Medikamente zu betrachten, ihnen allen gemeinsam seien und in einem direkten Verhältnis zu ihrer Wirksamkeit stünden. Diese Relation wurde illustriert durch Untersuchungen mit Tryptophan, bei denen aufgezeigt werden konnte, dass diese Aminosäure parallel zur Steigerung des Gehalts an aktiven Aminen im Hirn—durch die die Depression gemildert wurde—auch einen Anstieg der Amine im Gesamtorganismus bewirkte, mit dem eine Zunahme der Nebenwirkungen verbunden war. Eigentliche toxische Effekte sind hingegen präparat-spezifisch und haben mit der antidepressiven Wirkung nichts zu tun. Sie sind, wenn auch manchmal sehr schwerwiegend—zum Beispiel Lebernekrose—so doch selten und sollten im Zusammenhang mit der erhöhten Morbidität der Patienten, denen sie verordnet werden müssen, beurteilt werden.

CLASSIFICATION

A major breakthrough in psychiatry took place when Kline[1] and Kuhn[2] demonstrated that iproniazid and imipramine respectively were effective antidepressant agents. Since this time many other drugs have been introduced as antidepressants and pharmacologically they fall naturally into the imipramine group and the monoamine oxidase inhibitors. The pharmacological properties of these drugs are described more fully by Professor

TABLE 1.   The Similarity in Responses of a Depressed Patient to Two Different Drugs belonging to the same Pharmacological Group.

	1st drug	2nd drug	No. of patients
Response to two different MAO inhibitors	+	+	9
	+	−	0 $P = <0.01$
	−	−	7
Response to two different drugs of imipra-mine group	+	+	7
	+	−	1 $P = <0.01$
	−	−	4

Pletscher and Dr. Brodie. Briefly, the monoamine oxidase inhibitors are thought to exert their antidepressant action by virtue of their ability to inhibit the enzyme monoamine oxidase and thus increase the brain concentrations of monoamines of which noradrenaline and 5-hydroxytryptamine (5HT) are two important examples. The members of the imipramine group, on the other hand, resemble chlorpromazine structurally and in some of their actions, they do not inhibit monoamine oxidase and have little effect

TABLE 2.   The Inconsistency of the Responses of Depressed Patients to Two Drugs from Different Pharmacological Groups.

	Imipramine response	Imipramine no response
MAOI—response	5	15
MAOI—no response	15	30

on the overall brain concentrations of 5HT or noradrenaline but they potentiate noradrenaline, at least peripherally and, like the monoamine oxidase inhibitors they have a striking action in reversing the sedating effect of reserpine in animals. In clinical practice the response of a depressed patient to two different drugs belonging to the same pharmacological group, tends to be similar whereas the response to drugs from different groups is quite inconsistent. [3, 4] That this pharmacological grouping holds true in clinical practice is, of course, important not only in the management of patients but as a basis for clinical research (Tables 1 and 2).

INDICATIONS AND USAGE

There is general agreement that the antidepressants act against the endogenous elements in a depressive illness. The greater the neurotic or reactive factors, the less effective are the antidepressants.[5] They are, of course, quite ineffective in countering normal unhappiness secondary to some distressing event. This is not to say that antidepressants should be reserved for typically endogenous illnesses. Efforts to improve the environment or strengthen a patient's personality in a predominantly reactive or neurotic

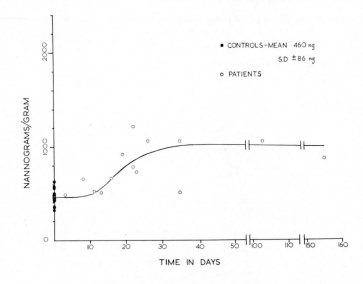

FIG. 1. 5-hydroxytryptamine concentrations in human mid-brain after oral administration of isocarboxazid.[6]

depression may be unavailing, yet the small improvement brought about by antidepressant therapy may enable the patient, with help, to overcome or adjust to circumstances which previously were insurmountable.

With both groups of antidepressants there is a latent period of approximately 2 weeks before the antidepressant effect becomes evident and the patient should be warned that improvement will be delayed. In general the earlier the beneficial effect the better the final outcome and the smaller the effective dose the better the result. It is usual to increase the dosage gradually but if improvement has not been attained after 3–4 weeks on a dose of, for instance, isocarboxazid 10 mg t.d.s. or imipramine 50 mg t.d.s. continuance of the drug or, further increase of dosage is unlikely to result in more than partial improvement. This clinical impression is reflected by the changes in the concentrations of 5HT in human brain which reach a maximum after

4 weeks administration of a monoamine oxidase inhibitor (MacLean *et al.*, 1964) (Fig. 1). If no improvement occurs a change of antidepressant to one belonging to another group is indicated, as a drug belonging to the same group, even if it is thought to be more potent, is less likely to be beneficial. Any improvement which is attained is more in the way of symptom relief than a cure, and the drug should be continued in a maintenance dose for several weeks or months until either a natural remission occurs or until the patient, now more capable of tackling their difficulties, has overcome or adjusted to whatever environmental stresses precipitated the depression.

WHICH DRUG, WHICH PATIENT?

That the antidepressants are not general euphoriants but act against a specific biochemical type of depression is suggested by the fact that a patient may be completely unchanged by one antidepressant yet respond dramatically to a drug from the other group. From a practical point of view it is obviously of great importance to be able to predict in any individual patient which group of antidepressant is likely to result in improvement and therefore which group to try first.

The problem has been approached from clinical, genetic and biochemical aspects and the present knowledge can be summarized as follows:

Clinical. Sargant has suggested that members of the imipramine group of drugs are the antidepressants of choice in the more typical endogenous cases of depression, whereas the monoamine oxidase inhibitors are indicated in the more reactive or atypical depressions. Most clinicians would agree with him,[7, 8, 9] though realizing that many typical endogenous cases respond best to monoamine oxidase inhibitors and many reactive or atypical ones to the imipramine group. West and Dally[10] and Alexander and Berkeley[11] have gone further and described a depressive syndrome which they claim responds specifically to the monoamine oxidase inhibitors. Features of this are the patient's good previous personality often with mild obsessional features, marked lassitude, and frequently the presence of phobic anxiety. The symptoms tend to increase as the day goes on and there is difficulty in getting to sleep rather than early waking. However, the more clinicians try to delineate in detail the sort of depressive illness which responds to one or other group of antidepressants, the more the subject becomes one of contradiction and controversy.

Genetic. Angst[12, 13] was the first to point out that patients tended to respond to imipramine in the same way as close relatives who themselves had been treated with this drug for depression. Pare *et al.* (1963) confirmed this similarity of response between patient and first degree relative[14] and found that in their patients it held with both the monoamine oxidase inhibitors and the imipramine group of drugs (Tables 3 and 4). Further work is being done to see if these results can be repeated. In the meantime we have suggested that there may be two genetically specific types of depression, the predisposition to which will, of course, breed true from one generation to another, and that one type will respond to the imipramine group of anti-depressants and the other to the monoamine oxidase inhibitors (Fig. 2).

TABLE 3. Family Correlations of Response to Antidepressants.[14]

Case No.	Drug	Response	Relation	Drug	Response
3	Phenelzine	+	Sister	Phenoxypropazine	+
13	Phenelzine	+	Sister	Parstellin	+
57	Amitriptyline	+	Father	Imipramine	+
236	Isocarboxazid	−	Father	Amitriptyline	−
	Imipramine	−		Phenelzine	−
243	Imipramine	−	Brother	Imipramine	−
	Isocarboxazid	−		Nialamide	−
			Sister	Imipramine	−
				Isocarboxazid	−
250	Isocarboxazid	+	Sister	Tranylcypromine	+
	Imipramine	−		Imipramine	−
300	Imipramine	+	Sister	Imipramine	+

TABLE 4. The Effect of Imipramine in Blood Relations.

+ = Responders, 0 = Non-Responders.
(Modified from Angst 1964.)

	Results of treatment of individuals			Results of treatment in pairs				Total No. of pairs	P
	+	0	Total	++	+0	0+	00		
Endogenous Depression									
Parents and children	38	1	39	20	1	0	0	21	0,05
Siblings	30	10	40	14	1	1	4	20	0,01
Distant relations	9	3	12	3	1	1	1	6	0,50
Total	77	14	91	37	3	2	5	47	0,001
Depression of Mixed Aetiology (e.g. Schizoaffective)	18	12	30	5	4	4	2	15	0,10

They suggest that the " imipramine gene " may be a more penetrating one and thus produce a more endogenous picture, the " monoamine oxidase gene " being less penetrating, only becoming manifest under stress and thus resulting in a more reactive or atypical clinical picture.

The difference between the clinical and genetic viewpoints can be illus-trated diagrammatically (Fig. 3). We suggested that it is the inherited bio-chemical abnormality, precipitated and made manifest by the patient's reaction to environmental stress, which determines the patient's response to one or other group of antidepressants. The other view is that it is a more non-specific biochemical disturbance secondary to genetic, personality and environmental factors in combination, which influences the response to therapy.

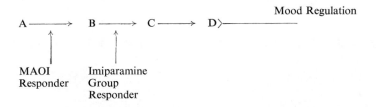

Fig. 2. Possible genetic types of depressive illness and their response to mono-amine oxidase inhibitors or the imipramine group of antidepressants.

Biochemical. Efforts to elicit biochemical differences between patients who do or do not respond to monoamine oxidase inhibitors have inevitably been hampered by the fact that whole body monoamine oxidase activity does not necessarily reflect that of the brain and monoamine oxidase inhibiting drugs may affect the brain to a different degree compared to other

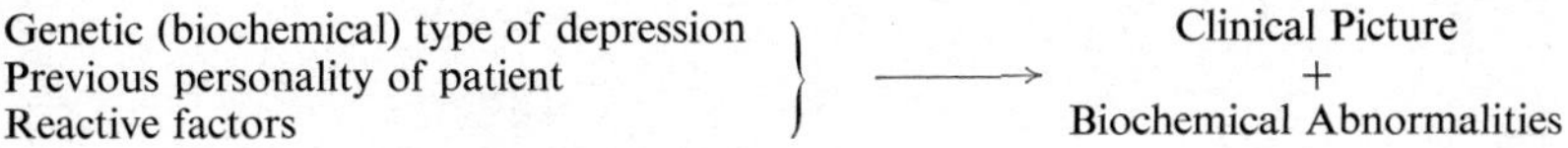

Genetic (biochemical) type of depression	Clinical Picture
Previous personality of patient	+
Reactive factors	Biochemical Abnormalities

Fig. 3. Factors influencing the clinical and biochemical picture of a depressive illness.

organs of the body.[15, 16] Furthermore, it is the changes in concentrations of brain amines which are thought to be important in the antidepressant action of these drugs and these changes do not bear a straightforward relationship to the degree of amine oxidase inhibition.[17] Nevertheless Tissot has reported that patients who subsequently responded to monoamine oxidase inhibitors had higher initial 24 hr levels of 5-hydroxyindoleacetic acid than patients who did not improve.[18] Recently he has been able to improve on this differentiation by giving an intravenous load of 5-hydroxytryptophan.[19] Curiously enough other equally careful workers have found completely opposite results.[20-22] Obviously these results have to be clarified but I do not need to stress how valuable such a laboratory test would be to clinicians however empirical it might be.

Research with imipramine is equally embryonic, but a promising line of investigation has been started by Kuhn and by Crammer in England, who are attempting to correlate the metabolism of the drug, as judged by urinary metabolites, with clinical response.

SIDE EFFECTS AND TOXIC EFFECTS

Side effects are common in most potent drugs and are part of their normal pharmacological action. They tend to occur to a varying degree in all the patients taking the drug, the higher the dose the more pronounced and frequent the side effects. They either remit spontaneously with continued treatment or disappear quickly when the dosage is reduced or the drug is stopped.

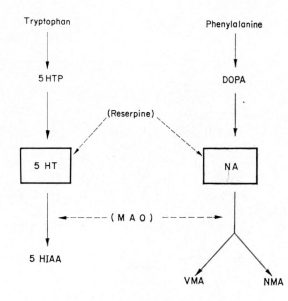

FIG. 4. The metabolic pathway of 5-hydroxytryptamine (and noradrenaline) and the site of action of monoamine oxidase.

In the case of the monoamine oxidase inhibitors the incidence of side effects seems to be closely related to the potency of the drug as an antidepressant, iproniazid being the most potent and causing most side effects, isocarboxazid, phenelzine and nialamide being less potent but showing few side effects and mebenazine coming somewhere in between. As has been mentioned above, the antidepressant effect of the monoamine oxidase inhibitors is thought to be due to their ability to inhibit monoamine oxidase which in turn results in an increase in the brain concentrations of various monoamines. However, the amine concentrations rise in other parts of the body at the same time, including the autonomic ganglia and the side effects are due in turn to this increased concentration of body amines. This was quite well illustrated in an investigation where, following Kety (Pollin et al., 1961), tryptophan was used in the treatment of depressed patients.[24] Tryptophan is the precursor of 5-hydroxytryptamine (5HT) and if used with a monoamine oxidase inhibitor would be expected to increase further the already high levels of brain and body 5HT (Fig. 4). On the other hand, when given to patients receiving imipramine, it would not be expected to

TABLE 5. The Effect of Tryptophan in Depressed Patients Receiving either Monoamine Oxidase Inhibitors or Imipramine/Amitriptyline.

	Much improved	Slightly improved	No improvement	Coincidental improvement	Total
Monoamine oxidase inhibitors	6	1	7	—	14
Imipramine/ Amitriptyline	1	2	6	1	10

have any effect as, of course, any 5HT formed would be rapidly metabolized by monoamine oxidase which is not inhibited by this drug. Briefly, it was found that tryptophan did indeed potentiate the antidepressant effect of the monoamine oxidase inhibitors but not of the imipramine group of drugs (Table 5). Furthermore, although it was well tolerated in those

TABLE 6. The Incidence of Side Effects when Tryptophan is Given to Depressed Patients already having Monoamine Oxidase Inhibitors or Imipramine/Amitriptyline.

	Nil	Hypotension/ postural hypotension	Nausea drowsiness	Hyper- reflexia musc. jact.	Perceptual changes
Monoamine oxidase inhibitors	6	14	5	4	1
Imipramine/ amitriptyline	8	—	1	—	—

patients receiving imipramine, patients taking a monoamine oxidase inhibitor got a marked increase in side effects, similar to those seen with the more potent monoamine oxidase inhibitors in full dosage (Table 6).

Another important issue is the effect of these raised concentrations of body amines when it comes to using drugs in combination or because of the effect of certain foodstuffs taken in the diet. These factors and their relationship to the hypertensive attacks seen, particularly with tranylcypromine, will be dealt with later in the symposium.

Toxic effects must be distinguished from side effects. Unlike side effects, they are not common to the group of drugs as a whole, they are not related to the clinical efficacy or antidepressant mechanism, they are not dose dependent and may come on at any time during treatment. Typical examples are the agranulocytosis found with etryptamine and the red–green colour blindness or even amblyopia seen sometimes with pheniprazine. One of the most important toxic effects is the hepatic necrosis found with some monoamine oxidase inhibitors. Iproniazid is recognized as being by far the most liable to cause jaundice, yet the best evidence available only gives an incidence of jaundice of 1/5000 and death for 1/20,000 patients treated.[25–27] The newer hydrazide-type antidepressants rarely give rise to jaundice and in

TABLE 7. Risks of Various Treatments.

	Serious toxic effects	Death
Iproniazid	1/5000	1/20,000
Tranylcypromine	? 1/50,000*	? 1/100,000*
Isocarboxazid	Negligible	Negligible
ECT	—	1/2000
Partial gastrectomy } for peptic	—	1/50
Pyloroplasty and vagotomy } ulcer	—	1/200

* See ref. 29.

the case of isocarboxazid not a single case of jaundice due to the drug has been reported in the United Kingdom and in the whole of the world literature up to September 1963, only two very doubtful and non-fatal cases were reported with this drug.

Obviously the antidepressants, like all drugs, should be used with care. I understand that over 250 million tablets of an antidepressant type—and this includes the amphetamines—are prescribed every year in the United Kingdom.[28] This is a fantastic amount and obviously it is wrong to use these drugs for minor mood changes. On the other hand it would be wrong to withhold one of these potent drugs from a seriously ill patient just as it would be wrong to withhold ECT if this were thought suitable. Again, the judicious doctor will usually prescribe the safer antidepressants initially and only turn to one with greater risks if the patient fails to respond. It is the doctor's job to assess each patient on his merits and to weigh the risks involved in any treatment he gives, against the morbidity of the condition he is treating. Taking into consideration the morbidity and the risks of the depression itself, or treatment with ECT, the complications of these drugs is a small price to pay for their undoubted value. This is certainly the case when one compares the risks of surgical treatment for a non-killing condition such as a gastric ulcer (Table 7). My own feeling is that when serious mishaps or fatalities are as uncommon as this, it is not so much the danger of the drugs but the skill and conscientious supervision of the doctor, or lack of it, which is important. Certainly an understanding of the pharmacology and mechanism of action of these drugs is essential if the clinician is to minimize their possible complications.

REFERENCES

1. LOOMER, H. P., SAUNDERS, J. C. and KLINE, N. S., *Psychiat. Res. Rep. Amer. psychiat. Ass.*, No. 8, 129 (1957).
2. KUHN, R., *Schweis, med. Wschr.* **87**, 1135 (1957).
3. DALLY, P. J., *Symposium on Depression*, Royal College of Surgeons, London, 1960.
4. DALLY, P. J. and ROHDE, P., *Lancet* i, 18 (1961).
5. DELAY, J. and DENIKER, P., *Canad. psychiat. Ass. J.* suppl. 4, 100 (1959).
6. McLEAN, R., NICHOLSON, J. M., PARE, C. M. B. and STACEY, R. S., to be published.
7. CRISP, A. H., HAYS, P. and CARTER, A., *Lancet* i, 17 (1961).
8. KILOH, L. G., BALL, J. R. B. and GARSIDE, R. F., *Brit. med. J.* i, 1225 (1962).
9. SARGANT, W. and DALLY, P., *Brit. med. J.* i, 6 (1962).
10. WEST, E. D. and DALLY, P. J., *Brit. med. J.* i, 1491 (1959).
11. ALEXANDER, L. and BERKELEY, A. W., *Ann. N.Y. Acad. Sci.* **80**, 669 (1959).
12. ANGST, J., *Psychopharmacologia (Berl.)* **2**, 381 (1961).
13. ANGST, J., *Arzneimittel-Forsch.* **14**, 496 (1964).
14. PARE, C. M. B., REES, L. and SAINSBURY, M. J., *Lancet* ii, 1340 (1962).
15. HORITA, A., *Toxicol. appl. Pharmacol.* **3**, 474 (1961).
16. McGRATH, W. R. and HORITA, A., *Toxicol. appl. Pharmacol.* **4**, 178 (1962).
17. GEY, K. F. and PLETSCHER, A., *J. Neurochem.* **6**, 239 (1961).
18. TISSOT, R., In *Monoamines et systeme nerveux central*, p. 169, Georg, Geneva, 1962.
19. BAREK, A., AJURIAGUERRA, DE J., BURGERMEISTER, J. J., REY-BELLET, J. and TISSOT, R., to be published.
20. VAN PRAAG, H. M. and LEIJNSE, B., *Psychopharmacologia (Berl.)* **3**, 202 (1962).
21. VAN PRAAG, H. M. and LEIJNSE, B., *Psychopharmacologia (Berl.)* **4**, 1 (1963).
22. VAN PRAAG, H. M. and LEIJNSE, B., *Psychopharmacologia (Berl.)* **4**, 91 (1963).
23. POLLIN, W., CARDON, P. V. and KETY, S. S., *Science* **133**, 104 (1961).
24. PARE, C. M. B., *Lancet* ii, 527 (1963).
25. FLOODY, R. J., DIXON, R. E. and MATTIA, V. D., *Dis. nerv. Syst.* **19**, 541 (1958).
26. POPPER, H. and SCHAFFNER, F., *Ann. Intern. med.* **51**, 1230 (1959).
27. GRIFFITH, G. C. and OBLATH, R. W., *Amer. J. med. Sci.* **244**, 593 (1962).
28. *The Times*, 23 May (1964).
29. *Brit. med. J.* i, 578 (1964).

PHARMACOLOGY OF
MONOAMINE OXIDASE INHIBITORS

A. Pletscher

Summary—Three different types of MAO inhibitors, i.e. hydrazine derivatives, phenylcyclopropylamine, and pargyline, are in clinical use. They cause a potent, long-lasting, irreversible inhibition of MAO and induce the following typical pharmacological effects on the central nervous system of animals:

Increase of endogenous monoamines, such as 5-hydroxytryptamine and catecholamines.

Enhancement of the monoamine increase and of the locomotor as well as the sympathetic stimulation due to administration of monoamines (e.g. tryptamine and tyramine) and their precursors (e.g. DOPA).

Counteraction against the monoamine decrease induced by monoamine releasers (*Rauwolfia* alkaloids and benzoquinolizine derivatives) and antagonism or reversal of their sedative effect.

These pharmacological actions as well as the psychostimulation in humans are probably connected with MAO inhibition. An increase of the free monoamines at the adrenergic receptors might be the biochemical correlate for the psychostimulant effect.

Résumé—Trois différents types d'inhibiteurs de la MAO sont en usage clinique. Ce sont des dérivés de l'hydrazine, de la phénylcyclopropylamine et de la pargyline. Ils causent une inhibition forte, irréversible et de longue durée de la MAO et sont à l'origine des effets pharmacologiques suivants sur le système nerveux central de l'animal:

Augmentation des monoamines endogènes, telles que la 5-hydroxytryptamine et les catécholamines.

Augmentation de l'accumulation de monoamines ainsi que de la stimulation locomotrice et sympathique provoquée par injection de monoamines (p. ex. tryptamine et tyramine) et de leurs percurseurs (p. ex. DOPA).

Atténuation de la diminution de monamines causée par des libérateurs de monamines (*Rauwolfia* alcaloides et dérivés de benzoquinolizine) et antagonisme ou renversement de leur effet sédatif.

Ces effets pharmacologiques ainsi que la psychostimulation décrite chez l'homme sont probablement en relation avec l'inhibition de la MAO. L'augmentation des monoamines libres au niveau des récepteurs adrénergiques pourrait correspondre sur le plan biochimique à l'effet psychostimulant.

Zusammenfassung—Drei verschiedene Arten von MAO-Hemmern, nämlich Hydrazin-derivate, Phenylcyclopropylamin und Pargylin, sind in klinischem Gebrauch. Sie verursachen eine starke, langdauernde, irreversible Hemmung von MAO und bewirken am ZNS des Tieres folgende, typisch pharmakologische Wirkungen:

Zunahme der endogenen Monoamine, wie 5-Hydroxytryptamin und Catecholamine.

Verstärkung des Monoaminanstieges sowie der lokomotorischen und zentral adrenergen Stimulation durch Monoamine (z.B. Tryptamin und Tyramin) und deren Vorstufen (z.B. DOPA).

J

Abschwächung des durch Monoaminfreisetzer (*Rauwolfia*-Alkaloide und Benzochinolizinderivate) verursachten Monoamin-Abfalls und Antagonismus oder Umkehrung ihrer sedativen Wirkung.
Diese pharmakologischen Wirkungen sowie die am Menschen beschriebene Psychostimulation stehen wahrscheinlich in Zusammenhang mit MAO-Hemmung. Die Zunahme der freien Monoamine an den adrenergen Rezeptoren könnte das biochemische Korrelat zum psychostimulierdenden Effekt darstellen.

Up to now, three classes of monoamine oxidase (MAO) inhibitors have been used in the treatment of mental depression (Table 1). These compounds differ in chemical structure and show multiple pharmacological actions which are due to various mechanisms, e.g. MAO inhibition, interference with other enzymes, direct action on pharmacological receptors. This presentation deals mainly with effects which seem to be the direct consequence of MAO inhibition and which concern the central nervous system.*

TABLE 1.

MAO-INHIBITORS

Chemistry	Generic name	Trade name
Hydrazine derivatives $R_1-NH-NH-R_2$	Iproniazid Isocarboxazid Nialamide Phenelzine Pheniprazine	Marsilid Marplan Niamid Nardil Catron
Phenylcyclopropylamine CH_2 ⟨⟩-CH-CH-NH_2	Tranylcypromine	Parnate
N-Benzyl-N-methyl-propargylamine CH_3 ⟨⟩-CH_2-N-CH_2-C≡CH	Pargyline	Eutonyl

1. EFFECTS ON MONOAMINE OXIDASE

The common property of the above mentioned drugs is their inhibitory effect on MAO, a mitochondrial enzyme occurring in numerous tissues. This enzyme catalyzes the oxidative deamination of primary and secondary monoamines like catecholamines, 5-hydroxytryptamine, tyramine and tryptamine into the corresponding aldehydes which are then further transformed into acids (e.g. vanillyl mandelic acid, homovanillic acid, and 5-hydroxyindolacetic acid) or alcohols (e.g. 3, 4-dihydroxyphenylglycol and 5-hydroxytryptophol). MAO inhibitors induce a potent, longlasting, and irreversible inhibition of this enzyme. Depending on the individual compound, concentrations of 10^{-3} to 10^{-7} M/l. *in vitro* and doses of 10–100 mg/kg *in vivo* have

---

* Detailed literature references are given in two recent reviews on MAO inhibitors.[1,2]

a marked effect. Due to the long duration of action, repeated small doses of the drugs cause an increasing degree of inhibition *in vivo* (cumulative effect).

The physiological role of MAO is not completely understood. The enzyme probably does not regulate the physiological content of monoamines of tissues like the brain. It seems to occur in great excess, because an increase in the cerebral monoamines can only be seen if the enzyme is inhibited to a

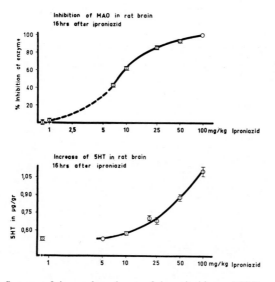

FIG. 1.   Influence of increasing doses of iproniazid on MAO activity and 5-hydroxytryptamine content of the rat brain.

Only with 25 mg/kg iproniazid i.p. the 5-hydroxytryptamine starts to rise significantly ($p < 0.01$), whereas MAO inhibition is almost 100 per cent.[3]

high degree (probably over 85 per cent)[3, 4] (Fig. 1). MAO might, however, exert a protective function by rapidly destroying the highly active sympatho-mimetic amines after their liberation from the storage depots (see below).

2.   PHARMACOLOGICAL EFFECTS IN ANIMALS

The mode of action of MAO inhibitors may be better understood if the present view on different monomine pools is considered first.

According to this theory, the monoamines of the tissue exist in a stored and in a free form. The free amines are biologically active and seem to be metabolized by the enzyme catechol-O-methyl-transferase. The stored amines are localized in special storage organelles (storage granules, nerve vesicles); they seem to be biologically inactive and protected from meta-bolizing enzymes. Part of the stored monoamines is probably localized close to the nerve endings, remote from the sites of metabolizing enzymes, such as

MAO. On nervous stimulation, noradrenaline can be released from this store without being inactivated and exert its physiological action on the adrenergic receptor. After its liberation at the nerve endings, the noradrenaline is inactivated mainly by re-storing (over 95 per cent) and to a minor extent by methylation in the 3-O-position by catechol-O-methyl

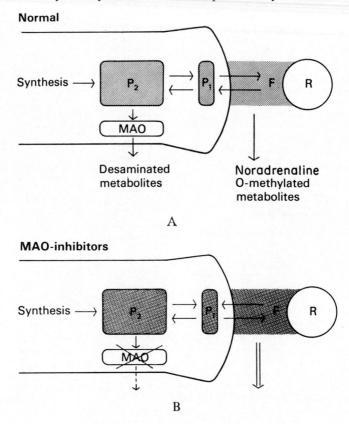

Normal

Synthesis →

P₂

MAO

Desaminated
metabolites

P₁

F

R

Noradrenaline
O-methylated
metabolites

A

MAO-inhibitors

Synthesis →

P₂

MAO

P₁

F

R

B

FIG. 2. Model of sympathetic nerve ending with the various monoamine pools and hypothetical action of MAO inhibitors on the amine pools.

P_1 = superficial monamine store, P_2 = deep monamine store, F = free monoamines, R = adrenergic receptor, MAO = monoamine oxidase.

transferase.[5-7] Another pool of stored monoamines seems to be situated in the vicinity of structures containing MAO (e.g. mitochondria). Noradrenaline released from this pool is immediately metabolized by this MAO and thus inactivated before it can exert a physiological effect[6, 8-12] (Fig. 2A). Although the evidence for this pool theory is mainly based on experiments with peripheral tissues (e.g. sympathetic nervous system, heart), it may be assumed that the central nervous system behaves similarly.

MAO inhibitors have three main pharmacological actions which are probably a direct consequence of MAO inhibition. They interfere with the metabolism of endogenous monoamines, with exogenous monoamines and their precursors, as well as with monoamine releasers.

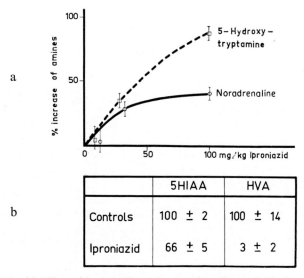

a

b

FIG. 3. (a) Effect of iproniazid on the noradrenaline and 5-hydroxytryptamine content of the rat brain.
    Ordinate: Increase of the amines in percent of controls, 16 hr after iproniazid i.p.
    Abscissa: Dose of iproniazid (mg/kg).
    The points represent averages ± SE.[30]
    (b) Effect of iproniazid on 5-hydroxyindolacetic acid (5HIAA) and homovanillic acid (HVA) of the brain.
    100 mg/kg iproniazid were administered i.p. 24 and 16 hr before sacrificing the animals. 5HIAA was measured in the brain stem of rats, HVA in the caudate nucleus of the guinea pig by spectrophotofluorimetric methods.[31] The figures are means ± SE and represent percentage values.

(a) *Endogenous Monoamines*

In various animal tissues, e.g. heart, brain, blood platelets, a high single dose of a MAO inhibitor causes an increase in endogenous monoamines, such as 5-hydroxytryptamine, dopamine, noradrenaline, normetadrenaline, which generally lasts for several days. Duration and intensity of action depend on the species and the individual inhibitor. In human tissues, e.g. brain and thrombocytes, a monoamine rise has also been observed after repeated administration of therapeutic doses of MAO inhibitors. Concomitantly, a decrease of desaminated metabolites, like 5-hydroxyindolacetic acid and phenolcarboxylic acids (e.g. homovanillic and vanillyl mandelic acid) occurs in brain (Fig. 3).

MAO inhibitors probably elevate primarily the monoamines in the pool which is close to MAO. In consequence, the free monoamines increase also, because an equilibrium of the amines in the different pools, including the free amines, presumably exists or because the amines might overflow after complete filling of the pools (Fig. 2B). This hypothesis is supported by the following findings:

Iproniazid increases the 5-hydroxytryptamine in the perfusion fluid of the isolated cervical ganglion.[13]

Nialamide causes an elevation of cerebral normetadrenaline subsequent to an increase of noradrenaline, indicating an overspill of noradrenaline from completely filled stores.[14]

MAO inhibitors in general seem to elevate the monoamine content not only in the particulate fraction, but also in the high speed supernatant of brain homogenates.[15-17]

The effects of MAO inhibitors on animal behaviour are not uniform, depending on species and individual inhibitor. Locomotor and sympathetic stimulation may, however, be seen especially after repeated administration of the inhibitors. The stimulation seems to parallel the increase of cerebral normetadrenaline indicating a rise of free noradrenaline.[14]

(b) *Exogenous monoamines and precursors*

MAO inhibitors increase the cerebral content of certain exogenous amines, such as tryptamine, tyramine, etc. After injection, these amines—unlike catecholamines and 5-hydroxytryptamine—penetrate the blood/brain barrier relatively easily. Their degradation in the brain is, however, impaired by MAO inhibition (Fig. 4).

MAO inhibitors also enhance the monoamine increase due to monoamine precursors, such as 5-hydroxytryptophan, 3, 4-dihydroxyphenylalanine (DOPA), tryptophan, tyrosine, etc. These amino acids penetrate into the brain where they are decarboxylated to the corresponding amines. These accumulate if MAO is inhibited (Fig. 5).

The functional effects of monoamine precursors, such as DOPA, 5-hydroxytryptophan, and of certain amines like tyramine, tryptamine, on the central nervous system are markedly enhanced by MAO inhibitors, especially locomotor and sympathetic stimulation, hyperthermia, tremors, etc. The central nervous stimulation parallels rather closely the elevated amine content in the brain. The stimulation is likely to be due to an excess of free monoamines acting on the adrenergic receptors. The amines probably " spill over " from the storage depots, which get overfilled because of increased supply and impaired metabolism (Fig. 6). A rise of some exogenous monoamines, e.g. tyramine, in the brain probably explains the central nervous effects of certain cheeses in patients treated with MAO inhibitors.[18, 19]

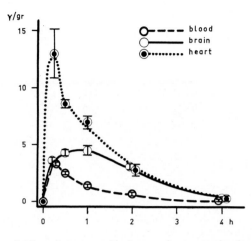

FIG. 4. Effect of 15 mg/kg tryptamine i.p. on the tryptamine levels in various tissues including brain after inhibition of MAO by 100 mg/kg iproniazid.

Ordinate: Tryptamine concentration in γ/g.

Abscissa: Hours after tryptamine injection.

The points represent means $\pm$ SE.

Without MAO inhibition, 15 mg/kg tryptamine do not cause a measurable tryptamine increase in the brain.[32]

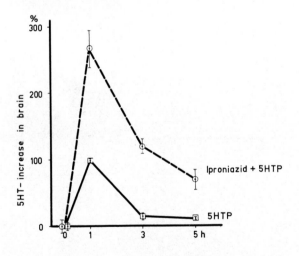

FIG. 5. Enhancement of the 5-hydroxytryptophan-induced increase of cerebral 5-hydroxytryptamine in rat brain by iproniazid.

75 mg/kg 5-hydroxytryptophan were injected i.p. alone or 16 hr after 100 mg/kg iproniazid i.p. The points represent means $\pm$ SE.[33]

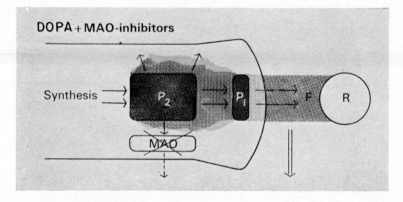

FIG. 6. Hypothetical action of exogenous monoamine precursors (e.g. DOPA) on the amine pools at the sympathetic nerve ending after MAO inhibition.

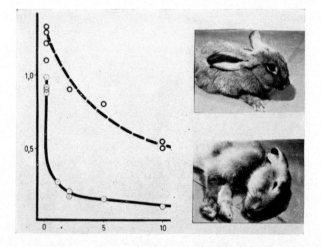

FIG. 7. Effect of monamine releasers on cerebral 5-hydroxytryptamine of mice and on behaviour of rabbits pretreated with iproniazid.

Curves: Ordinate: 5-Hydroxytryptamine content in γ/g.

Abscissa: Dose of reserpine in mg/kg.

Upper curve: Reserpine i.p. 10 hr after iproniazid s.c.

Lower curve: Reserpine alone.[34]

Pictures: Above: Animal treated with 40 mg/kg tetrabenazine (benzoquinolizine derivative) i.v. 16 hr after 100 mg/kg iproniazid i.v.

Below: Animal treated with 40 mg/kg tetrabenazine alone.[35]

(c) *Monoamine Releasers*

MAO inhibitors counteract the decrease of the total content of endogenous catecholamines and 5-hydroxytryptamine in the brain caused by monoamine releasers, such as *Rauwolfia* alkaloids and benzoquinolizines. The inhibitors also antagonize or even reverse some effects of the monoamine releasers on behaviour. Thus, after pretreatment with a MAO inhibitor, reserpine and benzoquinolizines no longer cause sedation, meiosis, hypothermia, and hypotension, but may induce stimulation, mydriasis, hyperthermia, and hypertension (Fig. 7).

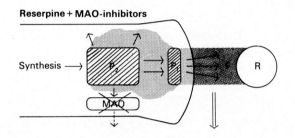

Fig. 8. Hypothetical action of monoamine releasers (e.g. reserpine or benzoquinolizine derivatives) on the monoamine pools at the sympathetic nerve endings after MAO inhibition.

The influence of MAO inhibitors on the action of monoamine releasers is probably due to a dual mechanism. At first, some inhibitors (e.g. iproniazid) seem to interfere with the release of monoamines from the storing depots. Therefore, a maximal depletion of the amine stores might be prevented, which possibly explains the attenuation of some actions of monoamine releasers by MAO inhibitors. Secondly, part of the monoamines released from the stores by reserpine is no longer inactivated because of inhibition of the main metabolizing enzyme MAO. This leads to an increase of the free monoamines and might be the reason for the central nervous stimulation which occurs after combined treatment with MAO inhibitors and monoamine releasers (Fig. 8).

3. PSYCHOSTIMULANT EFFECTS IN HUMANS

The mechanism which leads to the psychostimulant effects of MAO inhibitors in humans is still an object of controversy. The following principal difficulties complicate the problem:

(a) The pathophysiological function of monoamines, such as catecholamines and 5-hydroxytryptamine, in mental depression is not known.

(b) In laboratory animals, no spontaneous or experimental conditions are known which correspond exactly to human psychoses, e.g. mental depression.

(c) In man, investigations of the cerebral metabolism of monoamines are difficult to carry out. MAO inhibitors may affect the monoamine metabolism in the central nervous system and in the peripheral tissues differently. Therefore, conclusions based on measurements of the metabolic pattern of monoamines in blood and urine, as often carried out in humans, do not necessarily reflect the conditions in the brain.

(d) The quantitative action of MAO inhibitors on the cerebral mono-amine metabolism shows marked species differences. Conclusions concerning humans have therefore to be drawn with caution on the basis of animal experiments.

In spite of these difficulties, it may be assumed that the psychostimulant effect of MAO inhibitors in humans is causally related to MAO inhibition. Thus, the evidence is increasing that monoamines, such as 5-hydroxytryptamine and catecholamines, fulfil the requirements of neurohumoral transmitters. MAO inhibitors have been shown to induce marked MAO inhibition and monoamine accumulation in the human brain.[2, 20, 21] Furthermore, MAO inhibitors of different chemical groups (Table 1) may cause psychostimulation, whereas close chemical congeners, e.g. isoniazid, Ro 4-4602, not inhibiting MAO, but interfering with other enzymes, lack this clinical action (Table 2). It is reasonable to assume that the antidepressant effect is due to an excess of free monoamines in the brain. It has been shown previously that in *animals* procedures which presumably increase the free monoamines cause central stimulation, e.g. repeated administration of MAO inhibitors, injection of DOPA or reserpine after MAO. In *man*, tryptophan especially if administered after MAO inhibitors, shows psychostimulant effects (e.g. euphoria, loss of inhibition, and freeing of associations).[22-24] According to some authors, DOPA is of beneficial action on the dyskinesia and rigidity in patients with parkinsonism.[25-28] Free cerebral monoamines also seem to be of importance in the action of psychotropic drugs other than MAO inhibitors. Thus, thymoleptics like imipramine seem to increase the free monoamines of the nervous tissue possibly by inhibiting the restoring of monoamines released at the adrenergic receptors.[29] Reserpine and similar compounds, which are sedative and may even cause mental depression, on the contrary diminish the total and probably also the free monoamines in the central nervous system.

Whether catecholamines, 5-hydroxytryptamine or other amines are of primary importance for psychostimulation in humans remains to be elucidated. According to the recent trends of thinking, both types of amines seem to be involved, because a mutual interaction might exist in some pathways of the central nervous system.

In conclusion, good evidence exists that an increase of free monoamines in the brain might be the common denominator for some stimulant effects of MAO inhibitors on locomotor behaviour of animals. There are also reasons to assume that the same mechanism may be related to the psycho-stimulant effect of MAO inhibitors in humans. Due to MAO inhibition

TABLE 2. The drugs were administered parenterally to rats except in the experiments with DPN-ase (diphosphopyridin-nucleotidase), where they were added *in vitro*. For details see Refs. 1, 36, 37.

$$
\left.
\begin{array}{ll}
0 & \text{No} \\
+ & \text{Slight} \\
++ & \text{Marked} \\
+++ & \text{Potent}
\end{array}
\right\} \text{inhibition}
$$

Ro 4-4602 = N-(*dl*-seryl) - N' - (2, 3, 4-trihydroxybenzyl) hydrazine

INHIBITION OF VARIOUS ENZYMES
BY MAO INHIBITORS AND RELATED COMPOUNDS

	Monoamine oxidase (brain)	Decarboxy-lase (brain)	Diamine oxidase (intestine)	DPN-ase (liver)	Choline oxidase (liver)
Iproniazid	++	0	++	+	+
Tranylcypromine	+++	0	0		0
Pargyline	++	0	0		0
Isoniazid	0	+	+	++	0
Ro 4-4602 (Hydrazine derivative)	0	+++	+		

and a consequent delay of the metabolism, the stored amines are increased, which probably leads to a rise of the free amines and to their enhanced functional effect at the adrenergic receptors. Alterations of the cerebral monoamine metabolism seem, however, not to be the only cause for the psychostimulant effects of MAO inhibitors, because some of these drugs, like tranylcypromine, may also have a direct action on adrenergic receptors.

REFERENCES

1. PLETSCHER, A., GEY, K. F. and ZELLER, P., In *Progress in Drug Research*, II, p. 417, Ed. Jucker, E., Birkhauser Verlag, Basel/Stuttgart 1960.
2. PLETSCHER, A., GEY, K. F. and BURKARD, W. P., In *Handbuch der exp. Pharmakologie*, Erg. Band 19, Erspamer, V. Springer-Verlag, Heidelberg (in press).
3. GEY, K. F. and PLETSCHER, A., *J. Neurochem.* **6**, 239 (1961).
4. CHESSIN, M., DUBNICK, B., LEESON, G. and SCOTT, C. C., *Ann. N.Y. Acad. Sci.* **80**, 597 (1959).
5. HERTTING, G. and AXELROD, J., *Nature (Lond.)* **192**, 172 (1961).
6. POTTER, L. T. and AXELROD, J., *J. Pharmacol. exp. Ther.* **140**, 199 (1963).
7. HAEFELY, W., HÜRLIMANN, A. and THOENEN, H., *Brit. J. Pharmacol.* **22**, 5 (1964).

8. KOPIN, I. J., HERTTING, G. and GORDON, E. K., *J. Pharmacol. exp. Ther.* **138**, 34 (1962).
9. KOPIN, I. J. and GORDON, E. K., *J. Pharmacol. exp. Ther.* **140**, 207 (1963).
10. DAY, M. and GREEN, J. P., *Biochem. Pharmacol.* **11**, 1043 (1962).
11. GREEN, J. P. and FURANO, A. V., *Biochem. Pharmacol.* **11**, 1049 (1962).
12. CHIDSEY, C. A. and HARRISON, D. C., *J. Pharmacol. exp. Ther.* **140**, 217 (1963).
13. GERTNER, S. B., PAASONEN, M. K. and GIARMAN, N. J., *Fed. Proc.* **16**, 299 (1957).
14. CARLSSON, A., In *Adrenergic Mechanisms*, p. 558, Eds Vane, J. R., Wolstenholme, G. E. W. and O'Connor, M., Churchill, London, 1960.
15. GREEN, H. and SAWYER, J. L., *J. Pharmacol. exp. Ther.* **129**, 243 (1960).
16. WEIL–MALHERBE, H., POSNER, H. S. and BOWLES, G. R., *J. Pharmacol. exp. Ther.* **132**, 278 (1961).
17. SCHANBERG, S. M. and GIARMAN, N. J., *Biochem. Pharmacol.* **11**, 187 (1962).
18. HORWITZ, D. H., LOVENBERG, W., ENGELMAN, K. and SJOERDSMA, A., *J. Amer. med. Ass.* **188**, 1108 (1964).
19. TEDESCHI, D. H. and FELLOWS, E. J., *Science* **144**, 1225 (1964).
20. GANROT, P. O., ROSENGREN, E. and GOTTFRIES, C. G., *Experientia (Basel)* **18**, 260 (1962).
21. PARE, C. M. B., This Symposium.
22. LAUER, J. W., INSKIP, W. M., BERNSOHN, J. and ZELLER, E. A., *Arch. Neurol. Psychiat. (Chic.)* **80**, 122 (1958).
23. OATES, J. A. and SJOERDSMA, A., *Neurology (Minneap.)* **10**, 1076 (1960).
24. KETY, S. S., *Fed. Proc.* **20**, 894 (1961).
25. BIRKMAYER, W. and HORNYKIEWICZ, O., *Wien. klin. Wschr.* **73**, 787 (1961).
26. BARBEAU, A., SOURKES, T. L. and MURPHY, G. F., In *Monoamines et système nerveux central*, p. 247, Georg, Geneva 1962.
27. GERSTENBRAND, F. and PATEISKY, K., *Wien. Z. Nervenheilk.* **20**, 90 (1962).
28. FRIEDHOFF, A. J., HEKIMIAN, L., ALPERT, M. and TOBACH, E., *J. Amer. med. Ass.* **184**, 285 (1963).
29. THOENEN, H., HÜRLIMANN, A. and HAEFELY, W., *J. Pharmacol. exp. Ther.* **144**, 405 (1964).
30. PLETSCHER, A., *Schweiz. med. Wschr.* **87**, 1532 (1957).
31. PLETSCHER, A., BARTHOLINI, G., BRUDERER, H., BURKARD, W. P. and GEY, K. F., *J. Pharmacol. exp. Ther.* **145**, in press (1964).
32. PLETSCHER, A., KUNZ, E., STAEBLER, H. and GEY, K. F., *Biochem. Pharmacol.* **12**, 1065 (1963).
33. PLETSCHER, A. and GEY, K. F., *Psychiat. et Neurolog. (Basel)* **140**, 165 (1960).
34. PLETSCHER, A., *Experientia (Basel)* **12**, 479 (1956).
35. PLETSCHER, A., *Psychopharmacology Frontiers*, p. 395, Little, Brown, Boston 1957.
36. GEY, K. F., PLETSCHER, A. and BURKARD, W., *Ann. N.Y. Acad. Sci.* **107**, 1147 (1963).
37. GÖSCHKE, H., BURKARD, W. P., GREY, K. F. and PLETSCHER, A., *Med. exp. (Basel)* **8**, 256 (1963).

SOME IDEAS ON THE MODE OF ACTION
OF IMIPRAMINE-TYPE ANTIDEPRESSANTS

BERNARD B. BRODIE

Summary—Desmethylimipramine (DMI), a major metabolite of imipramine, elicits no obvious pharmacological effects of its own but, in doses comparable to those used to treat primary depression in man, prevents the syndrome of effects produced by reserpine-like drugs in rats. In larger doses, DMI " reverses " the effects of reserpine-like drugs to a unique hyperactive state (sponteneous excitation) in which rats fail to respond to external stimuli.

DMI counteracts the reserpine syndrome by blocking the cholinergic effects through a central action and by sensitizing central adrenergic receptors to the action of the brain catecholamines. The anticholinergic action antagonizes the muscle rigidity and the increased parasympathetic output and occurs whether DMI is given before or after reserpine. The sensitization of central adrenergic sites is observed only when the rats are pre-treated with DMI; this effect of DMI does not occur in animals which have been depleted of catecholamines by α-methyl-m-tyrosine. Furthermore, DMI counteracts reserpine sedation only if catecholamines are released rapidly by the reserpine-like compound. The importance of this rapid release is shown in studies with benzquinamide which, in DMI-treated animals, produces hyperactivity in doses that do not produce obvious sedation in normal animals and which release only 40 per cent of brain noradrenaline.

Résumé—Desipramine (DMI) un derivatif principal de l'imipramine, ne cause pas des effets pharmacologiques soimême, mais avec des doses comparable á la posologie dans l'homme il empêche les effets dans les rats des alcaloides de Rauwolfia et dérivés de benzoquinolizine. Avec les doses élevées, DMI produit un renversement de leur effet sédatif; il existe une stimulation locomotrice unique (" excitation spontanée "), quand les rats ne répondent pas á des stimulants externes.

DMI empêche les effets de reserpine parcequ'il cause une inhibition des effets cholinergique, par une action centrale et au même temps par l'augmentation des monoamines aux récepteurs adrénergiques centrals. L'effet anticholinergique attenue la rigidité des muscles et d'augmentation de la production parasympathique. Cet effet vient soit que l'administration de DMI est devant ou aprés la reserpine. La sensibilité des récepteurs adrénergiques centrals est observée seulement quand l'administration de DMI est le premier: cet effet ci de DMI n'arrive pas quand il y a une diminution de catecholamines dans les animaux causée pas le α-methyl-m-tyrosine. De plus, l'effet sédatif de reserpine est contrecarré seulement si les catecholamines sont liberées rapidement par une substance du type de la reserpine. L'importance de cette liberation rapide est vue dans les experiences avec la benzquinamide. Cette substance produit, dans les animaux, après l'administration de DMI, une stimulation locomotrice avec une dose laquelle, dans les animaux normals, ne produit pas un effet sedatif, et libere seulement 40 pur cent de la noradrenaline du cerveau.

Zusammenfassung—Desmethylimipramine, ein Hauptmetabolit von Imipramine, hat selber keine eigentliche pharmakologische Wirkung, verhütet aber, wenn gleich dosiert wie für die Behandlung von Grunddepression im Menschen, Wirkungen.

wie sie in Ratten durch reserpinähnliche Wirkstoffe auftauchen. In grösseren Mengen kehrt DMI die Wirkung von reserpinähnlichen Wirkstoffen zu einem einzigen überaktiven Zustand (spontane Erregbarkeit) um, in welchem Ratten nicht auf äusserliche Reizmittel reagieren.

DMI wirkt dem reserpinähnlichen Syndrom entgegen durch Blockierung der cholinergischen Wirkung mittels einer zentralen Tätigkeit und durch Empfindbarkeit der zentralen adrenergischen Rezeptoren auf Wirksamkeit des Katecholamin im Gehirn. Die anticholinergische Wirkung widersteht der Muskelsteife und der erhöhten parasympathischen Produktion und kommt vor, ob DMI vor oder nach Reserpin gegeben wird. Man bemerkt die Empfindbarkeit von zentralen adrenergischen Stellen nur, wenn die Ratten mit DMI vorbehandelt sind; in Tieren, welche durch α-methyl-m-tyrosin von Katecholamin entleert worden sind, kommt diese DMI-Wirkung nicht vor. Ferner wirkt DMI der Reserpin-Beruhigung nur entgegen, wenn Katecholamin schnell durch den reserpinähnlichen Wirkstoff befreit wird. Die Wichtigkeit dieser raschen Befreiung wird gezeigt in Versuchen mit Benzquinamid, welches in mit DMI-behandelten Tieren eine Ueberaktivität verursacht in Mengen, welche keine deutliche Beruhigung in normalen Tieren bewirken und nur 40% des Noradrenalin im Gehirn befreien.

INTRODUCTION

My interest in imipramine arose because of a naive belief that if a depressant drug produces sedation, an antidepressant drug should elicit stimulation. My feeling for the pharmacological fitness of things was upset by the fact that imipramine, a sedative drug in animals, was also a potent antidepressant drug in man.

If the rules of the game had been rigidly followed, imipramine would never have been discovered as an antidepressant agent nor, for that matter, would it have reached the stage of clinical trial. The animal screening tests then available could not have revealed this drug as a potential antidepressant. The drug elicits all the effects of a weak chlorpromazine-like drug. As seen in Fig. 1, the structure of imipramine is not unlike that of chlorpromazine. How did this sedative compound switch roles and become an antidepressant?

Drugs for mental disease are generally screened by means of behavioural tests in animals. In these tests the animal is treated in essence like a computer; the scientist programmes certain information into the animals; for example, they might be programmed for chlorpromazine. The more precise the programming, the less likely is the procedure to uncover drugs with a different sort of activity. This system of screening will give out only what is put into the system—another drug just like chlorpromazine.

The discovery of imipramine as an antidepressant emphasizes the value of a flexible approach in drug development. In the clinical testing of imipramine, the potential use of the drug was not precisely stated and instructions to the clinical investigator were purposely left vague. In this unbiased atmosphere it was possible for a brilliant investigator like Kühn to discover that imipramine was a new kind of antidepressant.[1]

For several years my good friend, Dr. Haefliger from Geigy, Basel, kept pressing me to carry out studies on the nature of the antidepressant action of imipramine. Frankly, I was not particularly interested. First, I did not see a clear way of studying in animals the antidepressant action of a drug that acts as a mild sedative in normal animals and man. Secondly, I did not believe the clinical reports. Finally, when the symptoms of endogenous depression were translated to me (from the German), my only thought was— no drug can possibly cure that! However, the sheer weight of optimistic reports as well as Dr. Haefliger himself finally wore me down.

How does one study the antidepressant actions of a sedative? Obviously, normal animals cannot be used; we must somehow set up a model depression in animals. But depression does not have the same meaning to a

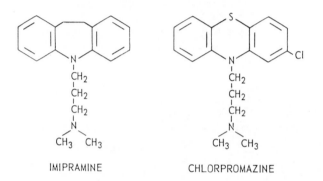

IMIPRAMINE   CHLORPROMAZINE

Fig. 1. Structural formulae of imipramine and chlorpromazine.

physiologist as it does to a psychiatrist and I did not wish to become entangled in semantic difficulties. I asked a psychiatrist friend to describe to me the symptoms of endogenous depression in a subject who had only recently acquired the disease. It seemed to me that I was listening to a description of the action of reserpine—even to its parasympathetic effects. We decided, therefore, that our model depression would be the syndrome of effects elicited by reserpine or reserpine-like compounds. I might say in passing that other psychiatrists chided me, perhaps rightfully, for comparing the depressant action of a drug with that of psychiatric depression. But it seemed to me that the psychiatrists must have also been deceived in the early days of reserpine when a number of elderly patients treated for hypertension ended up in institutions with endogenous depression. Some psychiatrists even refused to consider the depression as a drug effect and insisted that the drug had unmasked a childhood trauma.

Our first results with imipramine made us quite optimistic. As you know, reserpine not only produces sedation but activates, by a central action, the parasympathetic system, as shown by blepharospasm, meiosis, lachrimation, salivation, increased gastric secretion, and other parasympathetic signs which are blocked by parasympathectomy or ganglionic blockade.[2] Reserpine also reduces sympathetic activity but this is a peripheral action and can be accounted for by the depletion of noradrenaline from the peripheral sympathetic nerve endings. The preliminary studies showed that imipramine antagonized, apparently by a central action, a number of reserpine effects in rats and rabbits, including blepharospasm, hypothermia, diarrhoea, formation of stomach ulcers, salivation, and lachrimation.[3, 4] However, imipramine had no effect on reserpine-induced sedation.

We persisted in our attempts to determine whether reserpine sedation could be counteracted by imipramine. At times we were encouraged by results which seemed to show that imipramine had reduced reserpine sedation but the results were so erratic that I am sure we would have discontinued the problem had we not known that imipramine counteracts depression in man.

Fortunately, we had inbuilt in our programme a serendipity factor, an ingredient that I recommend with some reservations to the streamlined pharmaceutical laboratories of today—an animal caretaker who on occasion mixes the animals up a bit. One day he sent us rats that unbeknown to us had been receiving daily doses of imipramine for quite another kind of experiment. As a matter of fact, they were not even our rats—they belonged to Dr. Gillette and I can sympathize with his annoyance when he discovered that his animals had disappeared. Since we had no idea that the rats had been treated with imipramine, you may imagine our surprise when on administration of reserpine the animals almost literally climbed the walls!

PROOF THAT IMIPRAMINE ACTS THROUGH A METABOLITE

After promoting the animal caretaker, we tried to unravel these results by carrying out a time-response study with imipramine. The value of the dose-response curve has long been recognized in pharmacology but the value of the time-response relationship, especially when the response is related to the plasma or tissue drug level, is not so well recognized. When a pharmacological response is closely related in time to the presence of drug in plasma or tissues, it suggests that the compound itself is the active agent. If, however, the response is clearly unrelated to the plasma or tissue level, the possibility must be considered that a metabolic product might mediate the action of the drug (Fig. 2).

To determine the time-response curve, a number of rats were given a single large dose of imipramine (40 mg/kg i.p.) and at various times thereafter given reserpine. Imipramine readily enters the brain and in a few minutes the brain level reaches a peak and then declines exponentially. Reserpine injected 1 hr after imipramine elicits its usual sedation. However, when reserpine is given 3 hr after imipramine the sedation is markedly reduced. When reserpine is given 6 hr after imipramine, a frank excitation is elicited even though the imipramine level has declined to a low level. From these results it is clear that the antireserpine activity of imipramine is not directly related to its concentration in the brain.[5, 6, 7]

We made the not unreasonable assumption that if the antidepressant action were not attributable to imipramine itself, it must result from a metabolic product of the drug. In looking for such a metabolite, the pooled brains

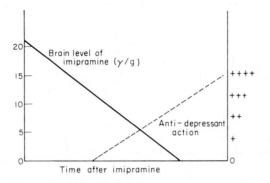

FIG. 2. Time-response curve for imipramine. An example of the type of response which is seen when a drug acts through a metabolite.

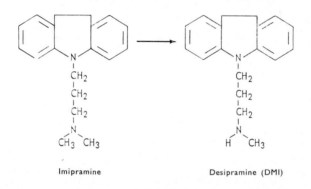

FIG. 3. Structural formulae of imipramine and desipramine.

from a number of animals, given imipramine 6 hr previously, were homogenized with water, the homogenate alkalinized and shaken with heptane. Phenolic material was removed by shaking the heptane phase with aqueous alkaline solution. Basic material still remaining in the heptane phase was returned to an aqueous phase by shaking with a small volume of buffer, pH 5·9, which extracts only minimal quantities of any imipramine that might be present. The fluorescent spectrum of this solution revealed material having characteristics similar to those of imipramine. Since the extraction procedure had been designed to eliminate imipramine as well as its phenolic

K

metabolites, it required no burst of brilliance to deduce that the metabolite was in all probability the monomethyl analogue of imipramine—that is, imipramine less one of the methyl groups on the nitrogen side-chain. We still had to identify the substance and the quickest way of doing so was to telephone Dr. Haefliger in Basel and inquire whether by any chance he had the monomethyl analogue sitting on the shelf. He did. Two days later the compound arrived in Bethesda and by the following day the metabolite was identified by gas and paper chromatography as the monomethyl analogue of imipramine.[8, 9] Chemically, the substance is called desmethylimipramine (DMI for short) and the generic name is desipramine (Fig. 3).

PROPERTIES OF DMI

We found that we had isolated an anomaly, since DMI, a potent anti-depressant, lacks pharmacological properties of its own. The pharmaco-logical profile of DMI, studied without reference to other drugs, gives no suggestion of its potent antidepressant properties and ordinarily such a substance would be abandoned to the pharmaceutical scrap heap. Unlike imipramine, DMI exerts no obvious sedation in rats even in large doses (40 mg/kg i.p.). Very large doses (60–90 mg/kg) may produce unco-ordinated hyperactivity that might be mistaken for an indication of its antidepressant action, when actually these signs are premonitory to convulsive seizures.

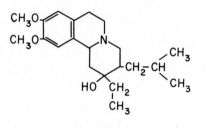

RO4-1284

FIG. 4. Structural formula of Ro 4-1284.

Dramatic effects of DMI are observed, however, when it is given to rats together with a reserpine-like drug. In these studies we used Ro 4-1284, a synthetic compound which has the structure shown (Fig. 4). This com-pound is one of a series of benzoquinolizines discovered by Pletscher and his associates[10] that exert typical reserpine-like effects. Unlike reserpine, its action comes on almost immediately and lasts only a few hours. DMI blocks or " reverses " the action of Ro 4-1284 much more rapidly and effectively than does imipramine (Table 1). Rats given Ro 4-1284 (15 mg/kg i.p.) 30 min after DMI (20 mg/kg) do not display the characteristic reserpine syndrome. Instead, they show a co-ordinated hyperactivity which is greatest after 1 hr and lasts almost 3 hr, about as long as the period of sedation produced by Ro 4-1284 alone.[11]

The rats given DMI together with Ro 4-1284 display the following behavioural patterns: Placed on top of a cage about 1 ft high, the animals ceaselessly circle the perimeter of the cagetop, peering over the sides and frequently leaping to the floor where they continue their avid " exploratory " behaviour (Fig. 5). Placed inside the open cage they almost invariably scramble over the sides. In contrast, normal rats placed on top of the cage move around and explore their surroundings for a few minutes after which

TABLE 1. Effect of DMI on the Reserpine-like Syndrome Elicited by Ro 4-1284.

| | Pharmacological effect | |
	Ro 4-1284	DMI followed by Ro 4-1284
Gross behaviour	sedation lack of motor activity hunchbacked posture	" alertness " motor hyperactivity
Muscle tone	increased	decreased
Autonomic	active eye closure meiosis bradycardia dilatation of ear vessels hypothermia lachrimation salivation diarrhoea	exophthalmus mydriasis tachycardia constriction of ear vessels hyperthermia no lachrimation no salivation no diarrhoea

they bunch together and groom themselves; rats given only Ro 4-1284 remain motionless and isolated from each other for 3 hr; rats treated with amphetamine dash erratically, not only around the perimeter of the box but crisscrossing it as well.

Placed on an elevated platform, the rats treated with DMI and Ro 4-1284 persistently poke their heads over the edge, each time stretching outwards a little more until finally they topple to the floor. Replaced on the platform, they repeat the performance despite a previous hard fall. By contrast, animals treated with amphetamine do not attempt the descent. The platform was only a few feet high but I have indirect evidence that the animals given DMI and Ro 4-1284 will jump from any height. One morning when I arrived in the laboratory, the animal caretaker whispered to me " Dr. Brodie, you can take it from me, the rats will jump from the seventh floor ". Since my laboratory is on the seventh floor, I decided I had not heard him.

In a treadmill, the rats treated with DMI and Ro 4-1284 turn the wheel continuously, about 300 times in 15 min, compared to about 15 turns for the normal animal. The animal plod on like automatons, rarely changing direction, hurrying but never running. In contrast, amphetamine-treated animals display erratic haste; at times they turn the wheel with a rapid burst of speed, then suddenly stop, often turn around and run the other way, and at times even attempt to climb onto the hub.

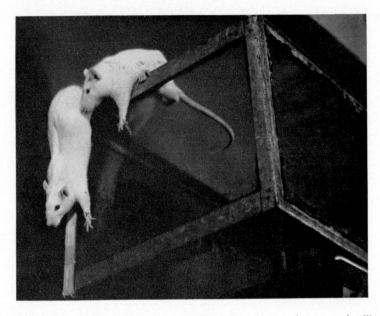

FIG. 5. Hyperactivity elicited in rats by desipramine and a reserpine-like compound.

After being deprived of food and water for two days, animals given DMI and Ro 4-1284 pay no attention to food or water, while untreated animals or animals given amphetamine eat and drink voraciously.

A conspicuous characteristic of the rats given the DMI and Ro 4-1284 is their seeming indifference to external stimuli. Unlike animals given amphetamine, they are undisturbed by violent shaking of the cage, by unpleasant noises, or by being touched. Also, they seem antisocial and appear oblivious to other rats. In their ceaseless prowling, when they approach other rats, they burrow under or climb over them as though the other rats did not exist. In contrast, rats given amphetamine courteously veer off to avoid a collision.

This unusual behaviour of rats given DMI and Ro 4-1284 left us with the

impression that the incessant activity stems from a " spontaneous excitation " rather than from an exaggeration of normal responses to external
stimuli.[11]

The effects of various doses of DMI on the action of Ro 4-1284 show that
2 mg/kg prevent muscular rigidity and parasympathetic effects (meiosis,
lachrimation, and diarrhoea); 4 mg/kg also counteracts sedation; 10 to

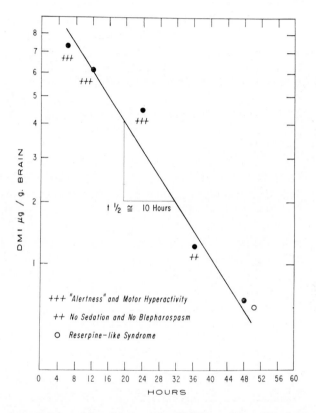

FIG. 6. Antagonistic activity of desipramine (DMI) on effects of Ro 4-1284 in rats
at various brain levels of DMI.

20 mg/kg reverses the effects of the benzoquinolizine and results in exophthalmus and an increase in spontaneous activity.

Figure 6 is a time-response curve which relates the effects of DMI to brain
levels of drug. In these studies rats are pretreated with a single dose of DMI
and then given Ro 4-1284 at various times thereafter. The results show that
the antireserpine effects of DMI against reserpine-like drugs are closely
related to brain levels of the drug.[11] In 24 hr at a brain level of about
4·5 μg/g, DMI still reverses the central effects of Ro 4-1284; in 36 hr at a

level of $1·25$ $\mu g/g$, the drug prevents but does not reverse the effects; and in 48 hr, when the DMI has almost disappeared, Ro 4-1284 now elicits the typical reserpine-like syndrome. Note that a similar sort of experiment has shown that the antireserpine effects of imipramine do not depend on its brain level.

Another peculiarity of DMI is unfolded by the discovery that DMI and Ro 4-1284 will not elicit sedation unless the drugs are given in the proper sequence. If DMI is given *after* the Ro compound, it no longer antagonizes sedation although it still counteracts the muscular rigidity and the parasympathetic effects produced by the benzoquinolizine. This was our first inkling that DMI might be exerting more than one action, but we will return to this later.

DMI counteracts the reserpine-like syndrome elicited by a number of drugs but has no effect on the sedation produced by barbiturates or chlorpromazine. Reserpine (2 mg/kg) injected intravenously into rats 30 min after treatment with DMI brings about the same unique pattern of behaviour elicited by Ro 4-1284 although the effects are somewhat less intense. Hyperactivity starts in 1 to 2 hr and lasts up to 24 hr, a time period similar to that of the sedative action of reserpine alone. The hyperactivity of the animals is punctuated by short intervals of repose (or perhaps exhaustion) after which they resume their forced marching. For the first 2 hr the rats show exophthalmus which in 4–6 hr changes to ptosis, presumably since noradrenaline has become depleted from the peripheral nerve ending.

Again, the sequence of administration is important. When rats are pretreated with reserpine, DMI blocks the parasympathetic effects and the muscular rigidity but not the sedative action. DMI-treated rats also exhibit spontaneous excitation after the administration of other reserpine-like benzoquinolizines, including tetrabenazine. Isoreserpine, a stereoisomer of reserpine that neither releases brain amines nor produces sedation, does not elicit hyperactivity in DMI-treated rats.

OF THE MECHANISM OF ACTION OF DMI

DMI does not inhibit monoamine oxidase, does not affect levels of brain amines nor interfere with the release of the amines by Ro 4-1284 or reserpine. It may be concluded, therefore, that DMI does not antagonize the reserpine-like syndrome by interfering with processes that metabolize or release brain monoamines.

Chlorpromazine in small doses counteracts the spontaneous excitation produced by DMI and Ro 4-1284. We considered the possibility that catecholamines might be involved in the antireserpine action of DMI and carried out experiments to determine whether DMI would still counteract the sedative action of Ro 4-1284 in the absence of brain catecholamines. Rats were given the synthetic amino acid, α-methyl-m-tyrosine which depletes the stores of brain catecholamines without affecting the stores of brain serotonin.[12, 13, 14] Twelve hours later the administration of DMI and Ro 4-1284 does not produce hyperactivity but instead elicits a typical reserpine-like sedation.

These results suggested that the antireserpine action of DMI might depend not only on the level of DMI in the brain, but also on the simultaneous release of catecholamines. Accordingly the effects of giving DMI and Ro 4-1284

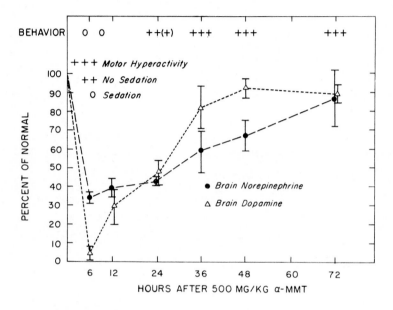

FIG. 7. Relationship between the antagonistic activity of desipramine on
Ro 4-1284 and the levels of brain catecholamine in rats.

at various times after the administration of α-methyl-m-tyrosine were related to the content of brain catecholamines. In 6 and 12 hr when the catecholamine stores are depleted, the administration of DMI followed by Ro 4-1284 produces a typical reserpine-sedation (Fig. 7). After 24 hr when the levels of dopamine and noradrenaline are about 45 per cent of normal, the combination of drugs elicits an almost normal degree of motor activity. In 36 hr with the dopamine level 80 per cent and the noradrenaline level 60 per cent of normal, the drugs now produce the characteristic picture of spontaneous excitation. These results suggest that the antireserpine action of DMI is conditioned by the amount of catecholamine released by the benzoquinolizine.

When studies from our laboratory showed that DMI is metabolized slowly in cats (half-life > 24 hr), we considered that this species was ideally suited

for studies of DMI action. The potential consequences of the cat's volatile
nature, DMI's long half-life and reserpine's protracted action (about 3
weeks) prepared us for the possibility that the animals might become
dangerously maniacal. However DMI and reserpine produced nothing more
than a yawn and a hearty sleep. Had we not observed the excitation elicited
in rats, we might well have given up the project at this stage. But I still
maintain that it is a mistake to give up a good concept because of a mere
fact. After all biology is not like physics or mathematics, and a theory does
not fall because of a single fact.

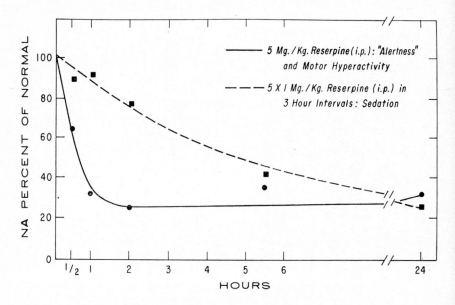

FIG. 8. Dependence of antireserpine action of desmethylimipramine on rate of
noradrenaline release. NA = noradrenaline.

We were biased enough to assume that something must be wrong with the
cat and our bias paid off. We found that in the cat, both reserpine and
Ro 4-1284 release brain noradrenaline: reserpine over a period of 6 hr and
Ro 4-1284 over about 4 hr, compared to the one hour or less in other
species.[15] This suggested that an important factor in the antagonistic effect
of DMI on reserpine-like drugs might be the rate at which catecholamines
are released. A slow depletion of brain noradrenaline over a period of 10 hr,
was then produced in rats pretreated with DMI by giving reserpine in small
repeated doses. These rats exhibited almost the same effects as animals
given reserpine without DMI pretreatment (Fig. 8). In contrast, pronounced
hyperactivity is observed in rats pretreated with DMI, in which noradrenaline

is rapidly depleted by giving a single large dose of reserpine. These results suggest that the antireserpine action of DMI depends on the rate of release of catecholamines, that is, on the brain level of free amines.

We then discovered another useful tool in benzquinamide, a recently developed benzoquinolize. In most species, this drug acts like chlorpromazine and does not release brain amines. In the rat however benzquinamide is deacetylated to the corresponding alcohol which elicits a reserpine-like action and releases brain amines[16] (Fig. 9).

Because of the formation of this deacetylated product, benzquinamide in doses that elicit almost no sedation, rapidly releases about 40 per cent of the brain noradrenaline and about 30 per cent of the brain serotonin. In

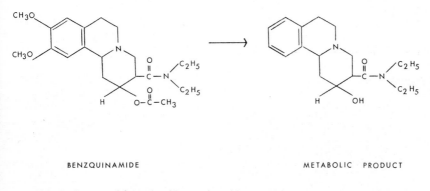

BENZQUINAMIDE   METABOLIC PRODUCT

Fig. 9. Structural formula of benzquinamide and its deacetylated metabolite.

rats pretreated with DMI, benzquinamide elicits a " spontaneous excitation " lasting $2\frac{1}{2}$ hr. From this result it is concluded that DMI will produce excitation in the presence of any drug that rapidly releases brain noradrenaline, whether the drug is sedative or not.

Thus, we have gone the full circle. Starting from the false premise that DMI acts specifically against the reserpine syndrome, we still managed to come up with approximately the right answer: that DMI produces excitation when given together with a drug that rapidly releases brain catecholamines. I find this sort of thing happening time and again in my laboratory, but I comfort myself with the thought that in biology a concept is never really wrong, the new concept is merely less wrong than the old one.

We then asked whether DMI would also potentiate the stimulant action of other adrenergic agents. DMI and amphetamine given to reserpinized rats produce a marked hyperactivity that lasts a number of hours whereas amphetamine given to these animals without DMI show hyperactivity lasting only a short time. DMI also potentiates the action of amphetamine in rats that are not pretreated with reserpine.

In addition, DMI potentiates the action of DOPA both in normal animals and in animals pretreated with reserpine. These results are consistent with the view that the antidepressant effect of DMI merely requires the presence of a sufficient level of free adrenergic stimulant in the brain.[11]

ACTION OF DMI IN RATS OF VARIOUS AGES AND STRAINS

The effects of DMI and Ro 4-1284 were studied in four strains of rats. DMI (20 mg/kg) and Ro 4-1284 (10 mg/kg) cause a marked hyperactivity in the Sprague–Dawley and Holtzman strains but not in the Osborne–Mendel and NIH Black strains. In the latter two strains, increasing the DMI dose

TABLE 2. Hyperactivity Produced by Desipramine (DMI) and Ro 4-1284 in Rats of Various Ages.

Rats were pretreated with DMI (20 mg/kg i.p.) and 30 min later were given Ro 4-1284 (15 mg/kg i.p.).

Age (weeks)	Weight (g)	Fraction of rats showing hyperactivity	Onset of hyperactivity	Duration of hyperactivity
2	25	0/6	—	—
3	40	0/6	—	—
4	75	0/6	—	—
5	120	1/9	2 hr	1 hr
6	160	7/9	1 hr	3 hr
7	180	2/3	1 hr	3 hr
8	200	7/10	1 hr	3 hr
9	240	8/9	0·25 hr	3·5 hr

to 40 mg/kg still fails to produce hyperactivity. Instead the typical spontaneous excitation is produced by increasing the dose of Ro 4-1284 from 10 to 15 mg/kg. In the Osborne–Mendel and the NIH Black strains the larger dose of Ro 4-1284 is needed to release brain noradrenaline at a rapid enough rate.

The age of the animals is an important factor in the action of DMI. Table 2 shows that in rats less than 5 weeks old, DMI and Ro 4-1284 produce no hyperactivity; excitation is produced only when rats are 6 weeks of age or older. These results are reminiscent of previous findings from our laboratory[17] which show that the brain noradrenaline level, low in newborn rats, increases slowly and in 6 weeks reaches 80 per cent that of the adult. Presumably, it requires 6 weeks for central adrenergic mechanisms to be fully developed in the rat.

SPECIES AND INDIVIDUAL DIFFERENCES

Whenever a therapeutic agent has been discovered by its effects in man and not from animal screening, it becomes of interest to determine under what conditions the drug could have been discovered in animals. Studies have shown that the action of some of these drugs would be difficult to test by the usual screening procedures because of their rapid metabolism in animals. At times these differences are so great that it seems a matter of pure luck that a drug is found clinically useful on the basis of animals experimentation. Let us see if imipramine and DMI could be revealed as a potential antidepressant drug in animals based on its ability to counteract and reverse the reserpine syndrome.

Based on results in mice, imipramine would be discarded forthwith. In these animals imipramine does not counteract reserpine sedation because the drug is rapidly metabolized and is not converted to DMI in appreciable amounts. Moreover the antidepressant action of DMI, itself, is not evident in mice because the drug is inactivated too rapidly.[9] Based on screening in rabbits, imipramine would again be discarded since this species rapidly converts the drug to inactive products. DMI itself produces only a minimal effect in rabbits since it is inactivated extremely rapidly in these animals.[9]

DMI or imipramine could not have been discovered in cats because in these animals reserpine releases brain noradrenaline stores much too slowly. Thus far, the rat had proved to be the only suitable animal, since this species readily converts imipramine to DMI and DMI has a relatively long half-life (9 hr). But even with this species we almost missed finding the active metabolite by not waiting long enough after injecting imipramine and we might well have missed it altogether had we used the Osborne–Mendel or the NIH Black strain.

Little published material is available on the metabolism and fate of DMI in man. We have determined the tissue levels of imipramine and DMI in a $2\frac{1}{2}$-year-old child who had swallowed a lethal dose of imipramine. Levels of DMI in most tissues were greater than those of imipramine indicating that imipramine is converted to DMI more rapidly than DMI is converted to other metabolites.[9] Another indication that man and the rat handle DMI in a similar way is seen from a report that patients treated with small doses of DMI and then given tetrabenazine or reserpine may become extremely excited.[18]

The rate of drug metabolism is a topic that should be of some concern to this group. A number of times today the merits of the double-blind test have been extolled. In the United States, the double-blind test has become a shibboleth and drug screening in man is not considered respectable unless it is also double blind. But a biologist sounds a word of warning when he hears that " double-blind " studies are carried out using fixed dosage schedules. The double-blind test involves a sound principle and is meant to separate factors such as variability of the disease process, bias, placebo effects, and so forth. But—and here is the rub—the use of this test implies that the drug is present in each subject in approximately the same amount in mg/kg. This might be true with highly polar drugs, substances which are not metabolized and disappear from the body at rates that are essentially similar among different individuals. In contrast, drugs that act on the brain, being highly lipid-soluble, undergo extensive metabolism at rates that are highly variable from person to person. Thus, the investigator applying the double-blind test in the belief that he is circumventing biological variability, may have substituted a situation in which the biological variability is vastly greater.

In my own experience the individual variability in drug metabolism can indeed be large. Studies of dicoumarol demonstrate that this drug shows a fourteenfold variation in rates of metabolism among different individuals.[19] Ethylbiscoumacetate shows equally wide variations in its rates in biotransformation,[20] in 4 hr the plasma levels of the first 8 subjects, all of whom received the same dose intravenously, were 0, 15, 35, 45, 70, 80, 130, and 160 μg/ml. Many other drugs are metabolized at rates that show wide variations among different individuals. It is evident that the use of double-blind screening can lead to utter confusion if, unknown to the investigator, the disappearance of the drug differs among the patients by several hundred per cent or more.

These individual differences in metabolism of drugs may be circumvented by relating the drug response to the plasma level instead of the dosage (in mg/kg). However, many drugs used in psychiatry are difficult to assay since they are highly potent and tend to accumulate in tissues. As a result, the plasma levels cannot be measured by present methods. New methods are urgently needed and I am hopeful that pharmaceutical firms will apply their skills to this urgent problem. At present, we have a number of extremely potent DMI-like compounds gathering dust in our laboratory. We have temporarily given up our interest in these compounds since it seems almost hopeless to screen them in man on any rational basis. How can you screen drugs against primary depression when they exert little or no obvious effect in normal man and you do not know whether the half-life is 30 min or 1 week? It is hoped that methods sensitive enough for the assay of these drugs in man will be available in the near future.

DISCUSSION

One of the confusing aspects about DMI is that it seems to exert two different actions against reserpine-like compounds.[11] In one action, also possessed by imipramine, DMI antagonizes muscular rigidity and increased parasympathetic activity. This antagonistic action is centrally mediated and occurs regardless of whether the DMI or imipramine is given before or after the reserpine-like drug. It is doubtful that reserpine stimulates central cholinergic pathways by a direct action and it has been suggested that it produces its cholinergic effects through a modulating action on these pathways, perhaps through free serotonin. It is not unlikely that certain types of parkinsonism might result from a disturbance of this modulation. Several reports indicate that imipramine is effective in patients with Parkinson's disease.[21, 22] No reports have appeared on DMI.

The second action of DMI is to antagonize and even " reverse " the sedation induced by reserpine-like drugs. This action requires the rapid release of stored catecholamines. In fact, studies with benzquinamide suggest that all that is needed for DMI to elicit hyperactivity is a rapid release of catecholamines in brain.

In retrospect, a marked change in activity produced by removal of a single methyl group is not surprising when one considers that most drugs that act on the nervous system do so by directly or indirectly affecting synapses. No argument is needed for the view that quaternary amines usually exert an action quite different from tertiary amines but we tend to forget that dimethylnoradrenaline has a quite different action from noradrenaline and that dimethylamphetamine has almost no central excitatory effects compared to amphetamine and methamphetamine.

DMI is not an isolated example of a secondary amine being a potent antidepressant while its corresponding tertiary amine is a tranquillizing agent. Sulser et al., in our laboratory,[6] first demonstrated that the antidepressant action of amitriptyline is mediated through a metabolic product, desmethylamitriptyline (nortriptyline). Bickel et al.[23] screened a total of 98 compounds by their antireserpine effect against the model depression described previously and showed that a number of DMI analogues show a potent antidepressant action in rats. In most instances, the corresponding tertiary amine shows sedation only. Antidepressant activity is not confined to the iminodebenzyl skeleton of DMI (Fig. 10).

For example, the CH_2—CH_2 that bridges the top of the middle ring can be replaced by CH=CH (iminostilbenes). Also, the C_2 bridge can be replaced by S (desmethylpromazine) or even omitted. Another important point is that the ring N can be replaced by carbon as in desmethylamitriptyline.

A particularly potent antidepressant agent by our test is desmethyltrifluopromazine. However, like most members of the phenothiazine series, it exerts a marked sedative effect. This fact is particularly pertinent since it focuses our attention on the narrow line that separates drugs which exert a chlorpromazine-like sedation from those that exert DMI-like antidepressant properties.

An analysis of the structure-activity relationships show that activity is restricted mainly to compounds having 3 carbons (unbranched) in the sidechain. In general, the activity is confined to secondary amines though the tertiary amines can exert a delayed activity through demethylation to the corresponding secondary amines. In contrast, the tertiary amines generally possess sedative properties.

An important question is whether the antireserpine actions of DMI are a reflection of its clinical action in depressed subjects. Thus far, clinical data indicate that DMI, desmethylamitriptyline, and desmethylpromazine exert beneficial clinical effects in primary depression.[24, 25, 26, 27]

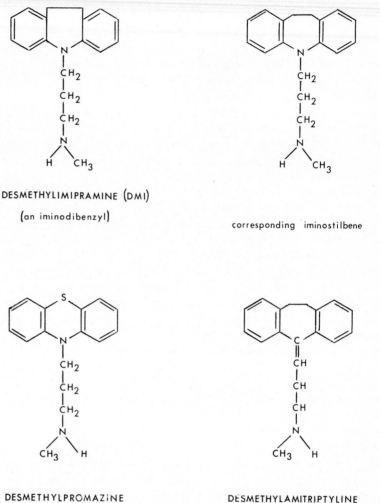

FIG. 10. Structural formulae of antidepressant compounds.

I have barely touched on the mechanism of action of DMI except to state that it may be associated in some way with central adrenergic mechanisms. A basic difference between DMI and other drugs used in clinical psychiatry must be borne in mind. In general, the latter act on the symptoms of mental disease by an extension of their pharmacological effects in the normal organism. DMI may represent a turning point in clinical psychiatry since it acts as an antidepressant only in the abnormal state. But this should be no great surprise since many of our most useful drugs for treatment of the non-mental diseases show their characteristic effect only in the abnormal state; antirheumatic agents, antiarrhythmic drugs, drugs for heart failure, to name a few.

Since DMI, a substance with little or no pharmacological activity of its own, elicits an antidepressant effect in depressed but not in normal subjects, it should stimulate the search for drugs that affect only the abnormal central nervous system. A challenging problem is how to set up abnormal states in animals. My own personal feeling is that this might be achieved by the use of drugs that provoke abnormal central nervous system activity. This approach might prove a welcome change from the current screening procedures; these have become frozen in concept and tend to ignore the existence of neural pathways. They are unlikely to uncover drugs that have a markedly different kind of activity.

Although DMI by itself exerts little action in normal animals, it interacts with many other substances. (1) It potentiates the action in various peripheral sympathetic receptors of administered catecholamines or catecholamines released at nerve endings. Based on these results, Sigg[28] first suggested that imipramine-like compounds may exert their antidepressant effects by sensitizing central adrenergic synapses. (2) DMI blocks the uptake of circulating catecholamines into storage sites at sympathetic nerve endings.[31] Since this is the mechanism by which the effects of the transmitter are terminated, it accounts for at least some of the potentiating effects of DMI in the normal animal. (3) DMI potentiates the action of catecholamines both centrally and peripherally in the reserpinized animal, showing that DMI must also exert some effect on receptor sites. (4) DMI not only interferes with the uptake of catecholamines but prevents their release by such agents as guanethidine, tyramine, and aramine.[32] (5) DMI *in vitro* interferes with the uptake of serotonin into platelets.[33] (6) DMI *in vitro* prevents the uptake of catecholamines into vesicles isolated from nerve endings or adrenal medulla.[34] (7) Our own work indicates that DMI potentiates the action of free catecholamines in the brain. It is this action that appears to account for the counteraction and reversal of the reserpine sedation. In addition, DMI potentiates the central stimulant effects of amphetamine-like compounds. (8) DMI, like imipramine may produce a marked potentiation of the action of monoamine oxidase inhibitors. This interaction can be severe and even fatal.[29, 30] This list could go on and on but I have mentioned these examples merely to indicate how complicated the effects of DMI may be. The results do suggest that DMI and similar compounds may affect certain micromembranes and that the nature of this interaction is a worthwhile fundamental study. But at present we can only say that DMI potentiates the action of catecholamines at adrenergic sites.

REFERENCES

1. KÜHN, R., *Schweiz. med. Wschr.* **87**, 1135 (1957).
2. BOGDANSKI, D. F., SULSER, F. and BRODIE, B. B., *J. Pharmacol. exp. Ther.* **132**, 176 (1961).
3. SULSER, F. and WATTS, J., In *Techniques for the Study of Psychotropic Drugs*, p. 85, Societa Tipografica Modenese, Modena, Italy, 1961.
4. COSTA, E., GARATTINI, S. and VALZELLI, L., *Experientia (Basel)* **16**, 461 (1960).
5. BRODIE, B. B., BICKEL, M. H. and SULSER, F., *Med. Exp.* **5**, 454 (1961).
6. SULSER, F., WATTS, J. and BRODIE, B. B., *Ann. N.Y. Acad. Sci.* **96**, 279 (1962).
7. SULSER, F., BICKEL, M. H. and BRODIE, B. B., In *Proceedings of the First International Pharmacology Meeting*, VIII, p. 123, Pergamon Press, Oxford, 1962.
8. GILLETTE, J. R., DINGELL, J. V., SULSER, F., KUNTZMAN, R. and BRODIE, B. B., *Experientia (Basel)* **17**, 417 (1961).
9. DINGELL, J. V., SULSER, F. and GILLETTE, J. R., *J. Pharmacol. exp. Ther.* **143**, 13 (1964).,
10. PLETSCHER, A., BESENDORF, H. and BACHTOLD, A. P., *Arch. exp. Path. Pharmak.* **232**, 499 (1958).
11. SULSER, F., BICKEL, M. H. and BRODIE, B. B., *J. Pharmacol. exp. Ther.* **144**, 321 (1964).
12. HESS, S. M., CONNAMACHER, R. H., OZAKI, M. and UDENFRIEND, S., *J. Pharmacol. Exp. Ther.* **134**, 129 (1961).
13. COSTA, E., GESSA, G. L., HIRSCH, C., KUNTZMAN, R. and BRODIE, B. B., *Ann. N.Y. Acad. Sci.* **96**, 118 (1962).
14. STONE, C. A., ROSS, C. A., WENGLER, H. C., LUDDEN, C. T., BLESSING, S. A., TOTARO, J. A. and PORTER, C. C., *J. Pharmacol. exp. Ther.* **136**, 80 (1962).
15. REVZIN, A. M., SPECTOR, S. and COSTA, E., *Int. J. Neuropharmacol.* **1**, 85 (1962).
16. WEISSMAN, A. and FINGER, K. F., *Biochem. Pharmacol.* **11**, 871 (1962).
17. KARKI, N., KUNTZMAN, R. and BRODIE, B. B., *J. Neurochem.* **9**, 53 (1962).
18. PÖLDINGER, W., *Psychopharmacologia (Berl.)* **4**, 308 (1963).
19. WEINER, M., SHAPIRO, S., AXELROD, J., COOPER, J. R. and BRODIE, B. B., *J. Pharmacol. exp. Ther.* **99**, 409 (1950).
20. BURNS, J. J., WEINER, M., SIMSON, G. and BRODIE, B. B., *J. Pharmacol. exp. Ther.* **108**, 33 (1953).
21. DENMARK, J. C., DAVID, J. D. P. and McCOMB, S. G., *Brit. J. clin. Pract.* **15**, 523 (1961).
22. MANDELL, A. J., MARKHAM, C. and FOWLER, W., *Calif. Med.* **95**, 12 (1961).
23. BICKEL, M. H. and BRODIE, B. B., *Int. J. Neuropharmacol.* in press.
24. BAN, T. A. and LEHMANN, H. E., *Canad. med. Ass. J.* **86**, 1030 (1962).
25. BRODIE, B. B., DICK, P., KIELHOLZ, P., PÖLDINGER, W. and THEOBALD, W., *Psychopharmacologia (Berl.)* **2**, 467 (1961).
26. KLINE, N., BRODIE, B. B. and SIMPSON, G., *Int. J. Neuropharmacol.* **1**, 55 (1962).
27. NODINE, J. H., SIEGLER, P. E., BODI, T., MAPP, Y. I. J. and DYKYG, R., *Pharmacologist* **6**, 180 (1964).
28. SIGG, E. B., *Canad. psychiat. Ass. J.* **4** (suppl.), S75 (1959).
29. DAVIES, G., *Brit. med. J.* **ii**, 1019 (1960).
30. SINGH, H., *Amer. J. Psychiat.* **117**, 360 (1960).
31. TITUS, E. O. and SPIEGEL, H. E., *Fed. Proc.* **21**, 179 (1962).
32. BRODIE, B. B. and BEAVEN, M. A., *Med. Exp.* **8**, 320 (1963).
33. SCHANKER, L. and FUKES, Unpublished.
34. This laboratory. Unpublished.

DISCUSSION

OPENER: ALLAN C. TAIT:

I feel that the best way to open the discussion on the treatment of depression, and particularly the mode of action of antidepressants is to present some of our data from Crichton Royal Hospital. This data may expand some of the observations in humans reported today by Pare and Pletscher.

Like other groups, we have been concerned for a number of years with looking for some correlation, in patients, between the biochemical and clinical effects of psychiatric treatments. Of these, drug therapy appears to offer the advantages of parallel study *in vitro* or in other species. Some seven years ago, feeling optimistic, I wrote[1] " Now, instead of passing a draught of electricity haphazardly across the skull, we have available compounds of known chemical constitution whose pharmacology can be studied experimentally ". This year, perhaps, I do not feel quite so optimistic: firstly because—in Dr. Brodie's words[2]—" variation between species, strains, and even among individual men, is fantastic "; and secondly because—and I hope this is not too provocative—the magic elixir of electricity remains the most potent weapon we have. Whoever finds the key to convulsive therapy may also find the key to both the major functional psychoses.

Meanwhile, we investigate drugs; mainly because with them we can use more techniques. The work I mention is essentially clinical, and to that extent inevitably untidy. In theory, it has the advantage of dealing with patients, in whom the meaningful change—and not any possibly imperfect analogue of it—is in fact taking place; and whatever we study is examined at the level of therapeutic dosage. In practice, professional ethics are apt to restrict our sampling techniques.

Some time ago we were looking at human platelet 5-hydroxytryptamine levels, reserpine being the obvious starting point. (As a by-product, before—and after—ECT studies showed nothing, as did insulin coma.) But it was reasonable also to screen whatever drugs became available for their effect on platelet 5HT in man. Amine oxidase inhibitors, of course, increased 5HT; but to our surprise, imipramine diminished it.[3] On standard dosage, we found a fall to 20 per cent of the pre-treatment level at the end of 3 weeks; the level thereafter reached some kind of equilibrium.

This observation seemed to deserve some pursuit. We found, *in vitro*, that concentrations of imipramine down to 0.5 $\mu g/ml$ caused some inhibition

147

of 5HT uptake. Later, Stacey[4], testing the effect of many pharmacologically active compounds on the uptake of 5-hydroxytryptamine, found imipramine by far the most potent, followed by cocaine and chlorpromazine. Long and Lessin[5] highlighted one of the difficulties I mentioned earlier when they showed that bovine platelets were vastly less sensitive to imipramine. This kind of finding, at any rate, encourages us to stay with patients.

We carried out a later screening[6] in vitro of imipramine and several of its analogues. In terms of 5HT uptake, imipramine was the strongest inhibitor, with amitriptyline next. Desmethylimipramine, desdimethylimipramine, and 2-hydroxydesmethylimipramine were less effective, and did not differ each from the other, or from desmethylamitriptyline. These differences were most marked at a drug level of 1 μg/ml, which we regarded, because of earlier work in vivo, as therapeutically obtainable. Chlorpromazine had no effect at 1 μg, but did have at 4 μg/ml: orphenadrine, a drug whose antidepressant properties have interested some of my colleagues for a long time, was ineffective at either concentration.

If the effect I describe has any relevance to therapeutic problems, it may be of interest that desmethylimipramine appears less active than the parent compound. Clinically in my hands it has not seemed clearly more rapid in action than imipramine; if any difference exists, it may lie in increased psychomotor activity, which was hinted at, I think by Poldinger, in the preliminary paper by Brodie and others[7] and echoed by Mann[8].

Another investigation of ours[9] showed that in vivo, the time course of 5HT fall produced by desmethylimipramine was indistinguishable from that caused by imipramine. At this time we were also concerned with the relation of plasma levels of desmethylimipramine to therapeutic response. At a dose of 150 mg a day plasma levels were around the 1 μg/ml mark I mentioned earlier. Clinically, we found a faint echo of Haydu's report,[10] working with imipramine, that the higher the plasma level of cyclodibenzyl compounds the less the therapeutic response.

This kind of comment—however inaccurate the example may be—indicates finally the goal one seeks in this type of clinical investigation. One chooses to hope that some chemical measure—here the amount of an amine, or the plasma level of a drug or of its various metabolites—may in its variation be related to clinical improvement. The difficulties at either end are great. The biochemical information available to us, in man, is peripheral. We measure what we are able to measure, and this may not be of primary significance for the drug's action. So pari passu with such estimations we have also to embark on studies designed to elucidate what underlying mechanisms may be involved; in our case, in some so far fruitless investigations of drug action on certain platelet enzyme systems.

On the other, purely clinical side, identification of patient change has its own problems, and this is particularly so in depression; an altogether damnable word, which sometimes seems to mean all things to all psychiatrists. The tedious nature of the estimates limits the number of patients studied; the fewer patients one has, the better one knows them; and the better one knows a patient the more one is unhappily aware of the many adventitious factors which may affect the course of his illness, perhaps more profoundly than the drug in question. In other studies some of my colleagues have tried to limit their field of vision by isolating one function for experimental study, namely, psychomotor activity. But, however inviting, such limitations may take us far from the heart of the matter.

In summary, our results point to an interference by cyclodibenzyl compounds with the uptake of amines. This appears consistent with the conclusions reached by Pletscher.

REFERENCES

1. TAIT, A. C., In *Topics in Psychiatry*, Eds. Rodger, Mowbray and Roy, Cassell, London, 1958.
2. BRODIE, B. B., In *Absorption and Distribution of Drugs*, Ed. Binns, Livingstone, Edinburgh, 1964.
3. MARSHALL, E. F., STIRLING, G. S., TAIT, A. C. and TODRICK, A., *Brit. J. Pharmacol.* 15, 55 (1960).
4. STACEY, R. S., *Brit. J. Pharmacol.* 16, 284 (1961).
5. LONG, R. F. and LESSIN, A. W., *Biochem. J.* 82, 4P (1962).
6. YATES, C. M., TODRICK, A. and TAIT, A. C., *J. Pharm. Pharmacol.* 16, 460 (1964).
7. BRODIE, B. B., DICK, P., KIELHOLZ, P., PÖLDINGER, W. and THEOBALD, W., *Psychopharmacologia (Berl.)* 2, 467 (1961).
8. MANN, A. M., *Canad, med. Ass. J.* 86, 495 (1962).
9. YATES, C. M., TODRICK, A. and TAIT, A. C., *J. Pharm. Pharmacol.* 15, 432 (1963).
10. HAYDU, G. G., DHRYMIOTIS, A. and QUINN, G. P., *Amer. J. Psychiat.* 119, 574 (1962).

OPENER: PETER DALLY:

Antidepressant drugs have been in general use for about 7 years. The confusion and contradictory views about the indications for using them that still prevail reflect our ignorance of the fundamental causes of depression and the lack of a universally accepted classification of depressive illness.

There seems to be fairly general agreement that hydrazine MAOI are most effective in depressive states where tension and anxiety are prominent (so-called reactive depressions), and that imipramine and other iminodibenzyl derivatives such as amitriptyline are better in the more endogenous* types of depression.[1, 2] However, both these groups of drugs seem to require reasonably mature or adequate personalities on which to act. Depressive states occuring in inadequate individuals or in children and adolescents do not usually respond to these drugs. Can this be related in

---

* These two types of depression being differentiated on clinical grounds and not on the presence or absence of a stressful situation.

any chemical way to the fact that children and many adolescents are very tolerant of large doses of amphetamine?

Some investigators have suggested that antidepressant drugs act only by virtue of a sedating effect.[3, 4] Certainly the hydrazine type of MAOI can be extremely effective in some states of anxiety, with or without depression.[1] They may be effective when given alone, but often their effect is greatly enhanced when combined with a tranquillizing drug. A combination of phenelzine and chlordiazepoxide, for instance, is highly effective in phobic anxiety states occurring in people with a good basic personality.[1] Giving imipramine alone to a patient with an agitated depression may make him more agitated. But when combined with a phenothiazine, imipramine may effectively relieve all depressive symptoms. Does the antidepressant act in such cases mainly by potentiating the tranquillizing effects? The tranquillizer given alone may have little or no effect. Is anxiety merely a symptom of depression? Or does the presence of severe anxiety interfere with antidepressant drug therapy (as it may do with ECT, for instance)? It is perhaps significant that patients with chronic tension and depression states, previously unresponsive to antidepressant treatment, may, after leucotomy, with subsequent relapse, respond to antidepressant drugs.

A good deal of publicity has recently been given to the possible dangers of combining an iminodibenzyl derivative with an MAOI. Since many patients respond specifically to one or other group of drugs, responding not at all or showing considerable intolerance to the wrong drug, it may be wondered why there should be any question of combining the two groups of drugs. But as Watts[5] recently wrote, there are patients, usually with a mixture of severe tension and depression, who only respond to this combination and with whom it is reasonable to accept the possible risks. So far as I know, all the reported disasters have occurred with imipramine and a MAOI. Sargant[6] has given amitriptyline and an MAOI to a large number of patients without serious side effects for several years, and it seems that this combination is sometimes very effective in otherwise refractory cases.

It seems unlikely that inhibition of MAO is the only mode of action of MAOI, although phenelzine, isocarboxazid and phenoxypropazine are certainly all comparable.[7] Iproniazid, however, is much more potent, both therapeutically and in side effects. Patients with long-standing tension and depressive states may recover on iproniazid and relapse whenever the drug is stopped or substituted by another MAOI. Tranylcypromine is not a hydrazine compound, although it is an MAOI, and the type of depression responding to it is more endogenous than reactive. An analysis of outpatients at Westminster Hospital responding well to tranylcypromine showed mild depression, manifesting itself mainly in complaints of bodily pain or discomfort and of extreme fatigue and exhaustion. Anxious patients who respond to the hydrazine MAOI may react badly to tranylcypromine and are liable to develop severe side effects, particularly headache. It is perhaps significant of the constitutional difference between endogenous and reactive depressions that all cases of headache resulting from taking MAOI (with or without cheese), seen over the past 2 years, have occurred in patients with reactive types of depression. Patients with endogenous depression seem to be able to tolerate MAOIs well from the point of view of side effects.

In spite of reports to the contrary,[8] there is a good deal of evidence that antidepressant drugs given concomitantly with ECT will often shorten the number of treatments needed.[9] But more important than this is the fact that some manic depressive attacks which were previously refractory to ECT given early in the attack will now respond if the patient is taking an antidepressant drug. When patients have recovered either as a result of drugs or ECT, it seems that in *some* instances antidepressant drugs continued during the period of wellbeing may be capable of preventing relapse. This is particularly valuable in cases of senile depression, where the prognosis was previously poor.[10] But it means that antidepressant drugs must be given for as long as the underlying depressive process continues, which may be years. It seems that provided depression has not become too " deep ", antidepressant drugs may be able to alleviate symptoms completely. But if depression is severe or response to drugs incomplete, ECT will almost always be needed. I think there is sometimes a danger that ECT may now be withheld for an unduly long time, or that an insufficient number of shocks may be given, the depressed patient then being left in a half-recovered state to await spontaneous recovery.

REFERENCES

1. SARGANT, W. and DALLY, P. J., *Brit. med. J.* i, 6 (1962).
2. KILOH, L. G., BALL, J. R. B. and GARSIDE, R. F., *Brit. med. J.* i, 1225 (1962).
3. HARE, E. H., McCANCE, C. and McCORMICK, W. O., *Brit. med. J.* i, 818 (1964).
4. HARE, E. H., DOMINIAN, J. and SHARPE, L., *Brit. med. J.* i, 9 (1962).
5. WATTS, C. A. H., *Brit. med. J.* i, 1114 (1964).
6. SARGANT, W., *Lancet* ii, 634 (1963).
7. DALLY, P. J. and ROHDE, P., *Lancet* i, 18 (1961).
8. KALINOWSKY, L. B., *Amer. J. Psychiat.* **120**, 944 (1964).
9. SMITH, A. C., *Brit. med. J.* i, 1184 (1964).
10. POST, F., *The Significance of Affective Symptoms in Old Age*, Maudsley Monograph No. 10, Oxford University Press, London, 1962.

GENERAL DISCUSSION

A. H. Crisp (*London*): Dr. Pare's results reveal an apparently significantly selective effect of different groups of antidepressant drugs on depressive illness in the same and different subjects including relatives. I am less sure of his interpretation of these results. They could, I believe, be due to a placebo effect or chance effect rather than a direct bio-chemical effect. I do not think he has used control groups or compounds in his studies. Intra-family discussions could be an important factor impinging on therapeutic effect in the study of probands and relatives. Could Dr. Pare please comment on this?

Derek Richter: I wonder if Dr. Pare would comment on the recent report of Japanese workers[1] that they have been treating manic patients successfully with imipramine. It seems possible that this might be due to some difference in diagnosis but, on the other hand, if there are genetic differences in the response that might be interesting. It seems possible that, for example, the ability of some individuals to demethylate imipramine might be relevant to the action in sedating manic patients.

C. M. B. Pare: Dr. Richter asked me about the Japanese workers treating mania with imipramine.[2, 3] Other workers[4, 5, 6] have classified not only imipramine but lithium too as mood normalizers, in other words, they correct the abnormal mood whether it is elevated or depressed. However, I understand that Dr. Hartigan[7] certainly is becoming doubtful whether, in actual fact, lithium does work in this way. Because of this I would certainly like to wait until these claims with imipramine are substantiated.

Replying to Dr. Crisp's remarks, I certainly accept that my results could be chance. I do not think, on the other hand, that it could be explained by a placebo effect because the proband and the relative usually had different drugs. Thus they would not necessarily expect similar effects. I certainly feel that the genetic aspect is worth further investigation and this is what we are doing. We all know that it does not work for every single patient.

Hannah Steinberg: I was very interested in Dr. Brodie's description of the behaviour of the rats given combinations of a reserpine-like and an imipramine-like compound; their syndrome of continuous moving about ("plodding on like automatons") seems strikingly similar to what Dr. Rushton and I have observed with some of the amphetamine-barbiturate mixtures which I referred to on p. 31. I wonder if Dr. Brodie would have found the same sorts of results as we did when we studied some aspects of this behaviour (exploratory activity and ataxia) by quantitative methods, and I also wonder whether we should find anything at all similar if we tried to analyse the mechanism of action of our mixtures in ways similar to his.

A. Pletscher: I would like to comment on the interesting remarks of Dr. Tait. Dr. Tait pointed out that imipramine-type compounds cause depletion of serotonin in the platelets and an inhibition of the uptake. I think that depletion does not have any bearing on what happens in the central nervous system. Many compounds have been shown to deplete serotonin from the platelets *in vitro* (for example, chlorpromazine, tyramine and many primary amines). Furthermore, with large doses of imipramine *in vivo* no depletion of the amines in the brain is found. So I do not think that the depleting effect in platelets *in vitro* reflects what will happen in the nervous system.

This is not so for the inhibition of uptake. We have good evidence that imipramine acts on the nervous system by inhibiting the re-uptake of amines. An example which I want to quote is the experiments on the isolated spleen nerve preparation which has been carried out in our laboratories by Dr. Hurlimann and his associates. If one stimulates the nerve of this preparation one gets, as you know, a contraction of the spleen. Furthermore, the output of noradrenaline in the perfusion fluid is increased. If the animals are pretreated with imipramine the contraction of the spleen on nervous stimulation is enhanced. Furthermore the output of noradrenaline in the perfusion fluid is very much enhanced too. This enhancement of the noradrenaline output in the perfusion fluid cannot be explained by inhibition of the degradation of noradrenaline for it has been shown that imipramine does not interfere with monoamine oxidase or on O-methyl transferase. It is known on the other hand that the noradrenaline which is released on nervous stimulation is mostly inactivated by re-uptake into the storage sites. We think that the most likely explanation is that this high output of noradrenaline is brought about by the inhibition of the re-uptake. This would tie in with what you find in the platelets. The inhibition of uptake is something which may reflect the mechanisms in the nervous system.

H. E. HIMWICH: In view of the fact that desmonomethyl chlorpromazine and desdimethyl chlorpromazine are weaker tranquillizers than chlorpromazine, both for patients and animals, I wonder whether or not desmonomethyl imipramine possesses weaker tranquillizing powers than imipramine. If so, perhaps part of the stimulating effects of desmonomethyl imipramine observed by you may be due to a comparative diminution of its tranquillizing action.

DR. BRODIE: The remarks of Dr. Himwich about the possibility of the effects of DMI being unmasked by the loss of the sedative properties are very pertinent and, actually, he has made quite a good point. A number of compounds of a tertiary amine nature are demethylated in the body. These include antidepressant compounds and some of the phenothiazines. Demethylation usually results in a less potent sedative substance. But the thing that makes your remark pertinent is that imipramine, at least in animal tests, blocks the action of desmethylimipramine, but only until such time that the imipramine concentration has declined to a level at which it does not elicit a sedative effect. If you give imipramine and desmethylimipramine together and then give Ro 4-1284, the excitation will be unmasked only when the sedative effect of imipramine wears off. Similarly, if you give DMI and the Ro compound and a little chlorpromazine, sedation will occur for an hour or two and then, when this wears off, excitation. I think that many of these phenothiazines inherently may have both actions but the sedative effect often masks the antidepressant effect.

The action of desmethylimipramine on membranes, as Dr. Pletscher said, has some component that prevents the re-uptake of catecholamines but this is not the whole story because in our experiments the factor of re-uptake was eliminated since by treating the animals with reserpine we had knocked out the binding sites. Thus, the antidepressant action of DMI does not seem to involve the uptake mechanism in our experiments. I suspect that perhaps the DMI-like compounds act on many kinds of membranes in the body. For example, DMI given even to reserpinized animals produces a powerful potentiation of the effects of the catecholamines although the factor of re-uptake has been eliminated.

An analogous situation may exist in another field. Dr. Born is doing some beautiful work in this country on agglutination of platelets. Reversible agglutination can be stimulated in vitro with substances like adenosine diphosphate or catecholamines. This effect can be blocked by a number of compounds including compounds like those that we have been talking about, imipramine, chlorpromazine, cocaine. This suggests that these drugs form a layer on a negatively charged surface and prevent the platelets from sticking. Since agglutination changes the permeability of platelets, the above-mentioned drugs may be said to interfere with permeability changes.

A similar type of reaction can be seen in the case of isolated mitochondria. Mitochondrial membranes normally undergo movements—almost like muscular movements—and if these are blocked by certain inhibitors, the mitochondria lose electrolytes, gain water and swell. You can prevent these events with the phenothiazines. On the other hand, once the swelling occurs, then the same compounds also prevent the restoration to normal.

DR. Tait mentioned that his blood levels of DMI are not related to clinical effects. I believe that he measured DMI in a plasma filtrate and the assay would include a number of metabolites.

One last point. Does Dr. Pletscher think that the monoamine oxidase inhibitors might exert some of their effects by inhibition of other enzymes?

A. PLETSCHER: I just want to confirm what Dr. Brodie said. I hope I did not make the impression that monoamine oxidase inhibition is the only mechanism of action of these compounds. As Dr. Brodie pointed out, many of these compounds interfere with quite a number of enzymes. For example, iproniazid interferes with diamine oxidase, thiamine oxidase, decarboxylase and non-specific oxidases in the liver, etc. Other MAO inhibitors have a different inhibitor pattern concerning these enzymes. This might be the reason why some clinical differences are seen between individual MAOIs as Dr. Dally mentioned. This may certainly also explain why they potentiate drugs which are not inactivated by MAO.

REFERENCES

1. AKIMOTO, H., Personal communication from the Department of Neuropsychiatry, University of Tokyo, Tokyo, 1964.
2. AKIMOTO, H., NAKAKUKI, M. and MACHIYAMA, Y., *Dis. Nerv. Syst.* **21**, 645 (1960).
3. AKIMOTO, H., *Proc. 3rd Meeting, Collegium Internationale Neuro-Psychopharmaco-logicum*, Munich, 1962.
4. SCHOU, M., *Brit. J. Psychiat.* **109**, 803 (1963).
5. SCHOU, M., *Psychopharmacologia (Berl.)* **1**, 65 (1959).
6. HARTIGAN, G. P., *Brit. J. Psychiat.* **109**, 810 (1963).
7. HARTIGAN, G. P., Personal communication, 1964.

SESSION IV

ANTI-ANXIETY COMPOUNDS

Chairman: WILLIAM SARGANT

USE OF DRUGS IN ANXIETY STATES

F. A. JENNER

Summary—The place of drugs in the treatment of anxiety has been considered. Their limitations have been emphasized but, as a part of the therapeutic approach, it has been suggested that drugs can play a useful role.

As the literature is full of contradictions one can only present personal recommendations and not a scientifically established approach.

The author considers that the diazepines are the drugs of choice in out-patient treatment of acute anxiety symptoms. When anxiety and panic are gross and intolerable, barbiturates and hospital admission still have a special place. In addition phenothiazines and meprobamate can be useful.

Phenothiazines are often helpful if prolonged treatment is envisaged as, in the author's opinion, the effects of the relaxant drugs are only temporary.

Résumé—On a vu la place des médicaments dans le traitement de l'anxiété. On a souligné nos restrictions mais en tant qu'une partie de l'approche thérapeutique on a dit que les médicaments peuvent avoir un rôle utile.

Etant donné que la littérature est remplie de contradictions, on peut seulement présenter des recommandations personnelles et non une conception établie scientifiquement.

L'auteur considère que les benzodiazépines sont les préparations de choix pour le traitement ambulatoire des troubles anxieux aigus. Dans les cas où l'anxiété et la panique sont très marquées et intolérables, les barbituriques et l'hospitalisation ont encore un rôle spécial. De plus, les phénothiazines et le méprobamate peuvent être utiles.

Les phénothiazines constituent souvent une aide précieuse si l'on envisage un traitement de longue durée, car d'après l'opinion de l'auteur, les effets des agents relaxants ne sont que temporaires.

Zusammenfassung—Es wurde die Bedeutung der Medikamente für die Behandlung der Angst besprochen. Wir haben unsere Vorbehalte betont, sind aber der Ansicht, dass Medikamente, wenn sie als Elemente einer umfassenderen Therapie eingesetzt werden, von Nutzen sein können.

Die Fachliteratur ist voller Widersprüche, so dass man nur persönliche Empfehlungen und kein wissenschaftlich fundiertes Konzept vortragen kann.

Der Autor ist der Ansicht, die Diazepine seien die Medikamente der Wahl für die ambulante Behandlung akuter Angstsymptome. In Fällen von heftiger Angst und Panik kommt der Verabreichung von Barbituraten und der stationären Behandlung immer noch ihre besondere Bedeutung zu. Ausserdem können Phenothiazine und Meprobamat von Nutzen sein.

Phenothiazine sind oft von Wert, wenn eine Behandlung über längere Zeit beabsichtigt wird, da nach Ansicht des Autors die Wirkung der relaxierenden Substanzen vorübergehenden Charakter hat.

---

* In this paper the word tranquillizer will be used to cover the *Rauwolfia* alkaloids, the phenothiazines, meprobamate and the diazepines. The words neuroleptics or ataractics will be used for the *Rauwolfia* alkaloids and phenothiazines, and the word relaxants for meprobamate and the diazepines.

DISCUSSION of the treatment of anxiety by drugs is bedevilled like other psychiatric problems by the difficulties of terminology. Though it is not appropriate to discuss nosology and the meaning of words here it is right to emphasize that without clarity in the use of psychiatric terms it is impossible to communicate very precise information.

The word anxiety is specially difficult because we all understand it from our own experiences, and it is not without meaning in everyday situations. There is, however, much to commend the view that despite our general ability to recognize anxiety in our patients when we see it, it is not always easy to distinguish it from depression or hypomania, etc. It is not, therefore, surprising if even with apparent care different results are achieved by different authors using drugs for *apparently* the same types of anxious patients.

According to many authors anxiety is to be distinguished from fear in lacking a well-defined object, but as far as drug treatment is concerned this differentiation is of little importance.

Drug treatment is a realistic, but alone is a clearly limited approach to the human misery of anxiety. If Scientific Therapy means knowing what one is doing, scientific drug therapy of anxiety should mean knowing that one is soothing but not understanding, unless one is also enquiring into the patient's psychodynamics. " One feels anxiety lest something occurs ",[1] and so understanding must be based on knowing what may occur. Usually something with special meaning to the patient.

Anxiety can be physiological or pathological depending on whether the degree to which the situation which has caused it, is such as would or would not do so in other people. The physiological anxiety for some awful ordeal ahead, e.g. criminal proceedings, bankruptcy, divorce, being found out, often warrants drug treatment if this will not impede appropriate reactions. In the same way, pathological anxiety deserves drug treatment if this will not obscure understanding, or if for reasons of economy of time the doctor has decided to forego further attempts to grasp the situation more fully. Further, it is warranted if the doctor really feels that though understanding people may be interesting it is difficult and does not help to change them.

As anxiety occurs as a symptom in almost any psychiatric syndrome, and in many organic states, the first step must be to separate the neurotic anxieties from those of schizophrenia and depression, the drug treatment of which syndromes is different, though the symptomatic treatment of the anxiety may be the same. This is also true of the organic states especially dementias and arteriosclerosis and parkinsonism. The patients in these cases are worrying lest their loss of control gets even grosser.

The drugs of use in anxiety states can be divided into, the primarily anti-anxiety drugs, those used for the accompanying insomnia, those used to correct the physical consequences of anxiety, for example, the low body weight, and those used to abreact the patient and so reveal the hidden dynamic factors.

The primarily anxiolytic drugs include the barbiturates, diazepines, meprobamate and the phenothiazines. Many other groups of drugs have been used but it is probably true that the above groups include the most appropriate drugs at present available for clinical purposes.

BARBITURATES

The mode of treatment must depend on the actual condition of the patient. In the absolutely incapacitating acute attack of anxiety, barbiturates are always effective if given in high dosage and the patient is put to bed to sleep for 4 or 5 hr. Amylobarbitone grs. 6, or pentobarbitone grs. 6, for example, will tide one over almost any emergency, but only until the next morning, when further aid must be made available. For prolonged treatment, phenobarbitone (grs. $\frac{1}{2}$–1 b.d.) can be useful as are other long acting barbiturates; it is not easy to recommend potentially dangerous drugs when other safer effective even if dearer agents are available.

The widespread use of barbiturates means that almost all doctors have a considerable understanding of their actions and it also testifies to their low toxicity. Barbitone was introduced into medicine in 1903,[2] since then 2500 barbiturates have been synthesized and about 50 used clinically.

The proper use of barbiturates for the relief of anxiety is difficult to categorize. It might, however, be wise to tend to limit their use to short-term treatment in hospital as a prelude to psychodynamic investigations or other treatments. They are very reliable if large doses can be used and the production of drowsiness is unimportant. They can, however, produce considerable confusion. Further, if large doses are used for a long time addiction can be produced and withdrawal phenomena are common, including epilepsy and delirium leading to states of exhaustion and even death.

Though drinking alcohol after barbiturates must be very common, there is enough evidence to indicate that this may, in certain cases, be dangerous and even fatal. Care should also be taken in cases of myxoedema, myasthenia, porphyria, respiratory disease and when renal or hepatic disease is present. The latter will lead to prolonged effects.[3]

Idiosyncrasies and skin reactions are rare, but urticaria, erythema multiform, exfoliative dermatitis and even the Stevens–Johnson syndrome have been reported. Agranulocytosis and other blood dyscrasias have been described.

The prolonged and excessive effects occasionally seen in patients after small doses, are usually hysterical reactions, and in these cases the psychodynamics of the patient should always be studied very carefully, before the patients are labelled hypersensitive by the doctor for his own sake. There is evidence, however, that nausea and vomiting can be genuine side effects with very small doses.

Barbiturates cross the placental membrane but are probably harmless to the foetus except at time of delivery.[3]

The fact that the barbiturates and other earlier sedatives are also hypnotics but that some more recently discovered drugs can control anxiety without producing sleep has led to the era of the tranquillizers.

The distinction between the minor tranquillizers and the ataractic drugs is not of such great importance in the treatment of anxiety. The consensus of opinion clearly rates the phenothiazines as the most important drugs in treating schizophrenia and so controlling hallucinations and other disorders of schizophrenic thinking. For treating anxiety the choice between phenothiazines, diazepines and meprobamate, etc., is more a matter of fashion. These drugs all compare well with the barbiturates in having lower hypnotic to sedative effect ratios.

NEUROLEPTICS

The evidence that the neuroleptics are often valuable in reducing anxiety as a symptom is considerable, of the relaxants is more controversial, though many consider them to be the drugs of choice. If the anxiety state is associated with symptoms which arouse any suspicion of schizophrenia, hypomania, toxic confusional state or other organic condition, it is probably wise to use a phenothiazine. There is also a case for their use when prolonged drug treatment is envisaged. The prolonged use of this group of drugs in patients is well documented and they represent the greatest contribution of pharmacology to psychiatry in modern times. Which phenothiazine to use is a question best left to the individual clinician who would probably be advised to stick largely to one such drug with which he becomes particularly familiar. On this ground alone chlorpromazine deserves special consideration because of the long and wide clinical experience already available.

The phenothiazines are being dealt with at some length by other contributors to this symposium and for that reason will receive limited attention in this contribution. For treating anxiety states six only might be considered, chlorpromazine, trifluoperazine, perphenazine, thioridazine, chlorprothixene, and promazine. For powerful action trifluoperazine, or perphenazine might be chosen, as a standard drug with a reasonable effect to toxicity ratio chlorpromazine can be used, where toxicity is feared thioridazine seems safer and a good choice, finally promazine can be used as a weak but useful drug in the elderly. It is difficult to define scientific criteria for the exact choice.

RELAXANTS

Personal experience in the clinical situation including some blind trials, makes it difficult for the author to accept the view that the relaxant drugs are ineffective. It must, however, be emphasized that apparently equally well controlled studies have produced apparently conflicting results. The possible causes for this are not difficult to surmise. The drug is only one factor in a complex situation. The fixed dosage regime may be designed to please the statistician rather than to help the patient. The cold mechanics of the rigidly scientific situation may increase the anxiety of the patient. The perceptiveness of the physician may vary as may his faith influenced often by subtle clues indicating the nature of the preparation through the apparent screen of the blind design. It is also difficult for psychiatrists to deny that as a group we are divided into those who want to believe and into those who do not want to believe. An interesting study of Uhlenhuth, Carter, Neustadt and Payson[4], for example, showed how one group of workers could get a significant, the other insignificant result for the same trial.

As mentioned above personal experience suggests that these drugs are indeed valuable in relieving anxiety. This relief may be only temporary while other mechanisms may induce recovery.

Experience also seems to indicate that though immediate benefits from the relaxants are often achieved the drugs are disappointing in long-term therapy. Many patients return week by week extolling the drug but still in obvious need of further help.

For reasons of economy, of space and time, only three drugs of this group will be discussed, meprobamate, chlordiazepoxide, and diazepam. The author feels that no other minor tranquillizer has as great a claim for consideration.

Meprobamate

The most widely used of the above group has been meprobamate, but it has now been mostly displaced by chlordiazepoxide and to an increasing degree by diazepam.

Many distinguished writers have selected for consideration a number of controlled trials of meprobamate which failed to distinguish it from a placebo. It is equally easy to quote controlled studies which show the opposite. A very short search of the literature revealed over sixty studies in which a placebo was used, the majority of which studies produced significant positive results. The clinician cannot adequately assess all this material, and quoting it fairly is not easy. Suffice it, therefore, to suggest that though the drug has severe limitations, from evidence in the literature the clinician is justified in using it for symptomatic relief of anxiety, headaches associated with neurosis and tension states including premenstrual tension.

The dosage of meprobamate should generally start at about 400 mg three times a day and if there is no response increase to 800 mg three times a day. If there is no response after a week on a high dose, another drug should be used.

Meprobamate is very safe, though rare examples of severe toxicity have been reported.[3] The toxic effects have included anorexia, vomiting, ataxia, delirium, parkinsonian tremors and muscular twitching, vertigo, impotence, blurred vision, irregular pulse, and hypotension. All these reactions are, however, rare. Hypersensitivity is also rare but anaphylactoid reactions have occurred, as have other allergic manifestations.

As with the barbiturates it is probably advisable to avoid alcohol, the effects of which are reported to be potentiated.

Addiction or mild habituation to meprobamate can easily be produced if treatment is maintained for too long,[5] but firm handling will, however, usually relieve this.

Diazepines

Rather like meprobamate, controlled trials of this group of drugs have shown conflicting results. They were introduced with too much publicity in the ordinary press, largely based on interesting animal taming results, but despite some disappointment in terms of the early and exaggerated claims, they have found a place in actual psychiatric practice, and one which has tended to replace that held previously by meprobamate.

Many consider this group of drugs to include the drug of choice for treating anxiety symptoms in various settings. Sargant and Dally[6] recommend a combination of chlordiazepoxide with phenelzine for reactive depressions. They include in this group most of those patients who have mixed anxiety and depressive features, and many with hysterical reactions. Paterson[7] combines chlordiazepoxide with imipramine, and ECT, for agitated depressions. Special claims have been made for chlordiazepoxide in offering relief in obsessive compulsive syndromes.[8] It may well be that this is more due to relief of the anxiety associated with attempts to avoid the compulsions rather than any ability to affect the obsessional symptoms themselves.[2]

As with meprobamate the diazepines seem to be either immediately effective, within two or three days, or else of little use. One is also impressed by the number of patients who claim great benefit but show little evidence of this. Experience in general also seems to show that even the sudden and dramatic responses which in themselves are so convincing, are difficult to sustain. Many might, therefore, agree that the diazepines are mainly for acute anxiety which can be managed in the out-patient department and, though helpful, are usually only a stop-gap which allows natural recovery to occur, time to attempt to manipulate the environment, or ease the burden in the early or critical stages of a psychotherapeutic approach.

The two major representatives of the diazepine group of drugs have so much in common that the selection of one rather than the other is often dictated by fashion and familiarity. On a weight for weight basis diazepam is more potent than chlordiazepoxide, but also more toxic. There has been more experience with chlordiazepoxide which might, therefore, recommend its use, but comparative studies[9, 10, 11] tend to show more favourable results with diazepam.

Jenner, Kerry and Parkin[12] felt 20 mg three times a day of chlordiazepoxide was excessive for most patients. They concluded that 10 mg three times a day was more appropriate. Maggs and Neville[13] felt that 10 mg three times a day was too small a dose, or the drug was not significantly effective in treating anxiety, the authors being unable to distinguish chlordiazepoxide from a placebo at that dosage. A consensus of present opinion might be that though 10 mg three times a day is a reasonable commencing dose 20 or 30 mg thrice daily is not unreasonable. Special care should be taken when prescribing for the elderly or debilitated when it is often wise to start with an initial dose of 5 mg, three times daily.

One can consider diazepam as approximately twice as potent as chlordiazepoxide, hence 5 mg three times a day is a reasonable dose; if the patient is elderly 2 mg three times a day can be used. There is little reason to fear doses of 15 mg three times a day, but drowsiness and ataxia may occur, and special care should be taken if the patient must drive a car.

The commonest side effects of the diazepines are drowsiness and ataxia. The drugs are, however, otherwise very safe. Hines[14], for example, reported a patient who took 1150 mg chlordiazepoxide in 20 min, and another who took 1600 mg in 24 hr, neither case required any treatment. The literature does, however, as with all drugs contain a long list of side effects which have been reported.[3] These include amnesias, hypomania, confusion, depersonalization, blurring of vision, dysphasia, dysarthria, hypotension, difficulty with micturition, loss of libido, various skin rashes, leucocytosis, agranulocytosis and eosinophilia. Though it is a doctor's duty always to be alert for any drug reactions, there are no special precautions required in treatment with the relaxants.

REFERENCES

1. FREUD, S., *The Problem of Anxiety*, Hogarth Press, London, 1963.
2. BLAIR, D., In *Modern Drugs for the Treatment of Mental Illness*, Staples Press, London, 1963.
3. MEYLER, L., In *Side Effects of Drugs*, 4th ed., Excerpta Medica Foundation Amsterdam, 1963.
4. UHLENHUTH, E. H., CANTER, A., NEUSTADT, J. D. and PAYSON, H. E., *Amer. J. Psychiat.* 115, 905 (1959).
5. ESSIG, C. F. and AINSLIE, J. D., *J. Amer. med. Ass.* 164, 1382 (1957).
6. SARGANT, W. and DALLY, P., *Brit. med. J.* i, 6 (1962).
7. PATERSON, A. S., In *Electrical and Drug Treatments in Psychiatry*, Elsevier, Amsterdam, 1963.
8. TOBIN, J. M., BIRD, I. F. and BOYLE, D. E., *Dis. nerv. Syst.* 21, suppl. 11 (1960–).
9. KERRY, R. J. and JENNER, F. A., *Psychopharmacologia (Berl.)* 3, 302 (1962).
10. DANEMAN, E. A., *J. med. Ass. Ga.* 53, 55 (1964).

M

11. DARLING, H. F., *Dis. nerv. Syst.* **24**, 501 (1963).
12. JENNER, F. A., KERRY, R. J. and PARKIN, D., *J. ment. Sci.* **107**, 575 and 583 (1961).
13. MAGGS, R. and NEVILLE, R., *Brit. J. Psychiat.* **110**, 540 (1964).
14. HINES, L. R., *Curr. ther. Res.* **2**, 227 (1960).

MODE OF ACTION OF
ANTI-ANXIETY COMPOUNDS*

GEORGE A. HEISE

Summary—Meprobamate and chlordiazepoxide are members of a distinct class of anti-anxiety drugs that act alike in pharmacological screening and operant conditioning situations, and in electrophysiological studies of the central nervous system. Phenobarbitone acts like meprobamate and chlordiazepoxide in most of the behavioural experiments, but has quite different effects on the central nervous system. Effects of the phenothiazines and of other barbiturates on behaviour and on the central nervous system are qualitatively different from those of the anti-anxiety drugs.

No consistent mechanism of action can be discerned in the variety of complex types of behaviours affected by the anti-anxiety drugs in various tests. All the anti-anxiety drugs are anti-convulsants and muscle relaxants, " tame " or reduce fighting in aggressive animals, and increase the amount of food eaten by deprived animals. They also produce a relatively large proportion of " gap responses " in discrete-trial " trace " avoidance, and increase response rate in certain operant schedules in which the responses are widely spaced. However, experiments on response-contingent punishment (" conflict ") suggest that the anti-anxiety drugs may specifically attenuate passive avoidance behaviour (learning *not* to respond). This conclusion is compatible with the clinical use of the drugs for " anxious " patients and with a possible site of drug action in the limbic system.

Résumé—Le méprobamate et le chlordiazépoxide font partie d'une classe distincte d'agents anxiolytiques qui agissent de façon semblable dans les examens pharmacologiques de routine et les tests de conditionnement, et dans les études neurophysiologiques du système nerveux central. Le phénobarbital agit comme le méprobamate et le chlordiazépoxide dans la plupart des expériences sur le comportement, mais il a des effets complètement différents sur le système nerveux central. Les effets des phénothiazines et ceux des barbituriques sur le comportement et sur le système nerveux central diffèrent qualitativement de ceux des agents anxiolytiques. Vu la variété des comportements complexes affectés par les agents anxiolytiques dans les divers tests, on ne peut discerner de mécanisme d'action uniforme. Tous les anxiolytiques sont des anti-convulsivants et des myorelaxants: ils " apprivoisent " ou réduisent l'humeur batailleuse chez les animaux agressifs et accroissent la quantité de nourriture absorbée par les animaux soumis au jeûne. Ils produisent aussi une proportion relativement importante de réponses pendant la phase de silence dans le test d'évitement léger et augmentent le pourcentage de réponse dans certaines épreuves caractérisées par un grand intervalle entre les réponses. Cependant, des expériences conflictogènes suggèrent la possibilité pour les médicaments anxiolytiques d'atténuer d'une manière spécifique le comportement passif d'évitement (l'animal apprend à *ne pas* répondre). Cette conclusion est compatible avec l'utilisation clinique des médicaments pour les malades " anxieux " et avec un éventuel point d'impact dans le système limbique.

---

* Preparation of this paper was supported by a grant, PHS MH 06997-02, from the National Institute of Mental Health to Indiana University.

Zusammenfassung—Meprobamat und Chlordiazepoxyd gehören einer deutlich abgrenzbaren Gruppe von angstlösenden Medikamenten an, die in pharmakologischen und Verhaltenstests sowie in elektrophysiologischen Untersuchungen des ZNS zu ähnlichen Ergebnissen führen. Phenobarbital wirkt bei den meisten Verhaltensstudien gleich wie Meprobamat und Chlordiazepoxyd, hat aber ganz andere Auswirkungen auf das ZNS. Der Effekt von Phenothiazin und von anderen Barbituraten als Phenobarbital auf Verhalten und ZNS sind qualitativ von denen der Anxiolytica verschieden.

Aus der Vielfalt komplexer Verhaltensweisen, die in verschiedenen Tests durch Anxiolytica beeinflusst werden, kann kein einheitlicher Wirkungsmechanismus abgeleitet werden. Alle angstlösenden Substanzen wirken anti-konvulsiv und muskelrelaxierend, sie " zähmen " wilde Tiere oder vermindern ihre Aggressivität; und erhöhen die Futtermenge, die von hungernden Tieren aufgenommen wird. Sie bewirken auch einen relativ hohen Prozentsatz an " Intervall-Reaktionen " bei Tieren, die gelernt hatten, auf ein Signal hin einen elektrischen Schlag zu vermeiden und erhöhen die Reaktionsquoten bei Versuchsanordnungen, bei denen die verlangten Reaktionen zeitlich weit auseinanderliegen. Allerdings weisen sog. Konfliktversuche, bei denen die Reaktion eine Strafe auslösen kann, darauf hin, dass Anxiolytica die Verhaltensweise des passiven Vermeidens (Nicht-reagieren-Lernens) spezifisch beeinträchtigt. Diese Schlussfolgerung ist vereinbar mit der klinischen Verwendung dieser Medikamente bei "ängstlichen" Patienten und mit der Möglichkeit ihres Angriffspunkts im limbischen System.

INQUIRY into the mode of action of anti-anxiety drugs raises the following questions:

1. Do the anti-anxiety drugs constitute a separate functional class: do they have effects that are similar for the drugs within the class but are different from the effects of other classes such as the " major tranquillizers " or sedative-hypnotics?

2. What are the behavioural or physiological mechanisms by which common effects (if any) of the anti-anxiety drugs are produced? Can these mechanisms be identified as " anti-anxiety "?

3. What kinds of extrapolations can be made to humans from the findings of animal research on the properties and mechanisms of action of anti-anxiety drugs?

By " anti-anxiety " drugs, we mean those drugs that clinicians use to treat " anxious " patients. However, the clinician's definition of " anxiety " is hardly precise, consisting of an intuitive combination of subjective impressions (feelings of tension, guilt, apprehension, dependency, and loss of confidence) and more-or-less objective observations of restlessness and autonomic symptoms. But, paradoxically, even though clinicians are unclear as to what " anxiety " is, they, nevertheless, agree on which drugs are the *anti*-anxiety drugs. The anti-anxiety drugs are also called " minor tranquillizers " because they are used typically for the relatively mild disorders of the non-psychotic, or neurotic. Clinicians believe that the minor tranquillizers have different effects from the " major tranquillizers ", such as the phenothiazines. The major tranquillizers are given chiefly to psychotics and are not usually regarded as very effective against anxiety. The clinician typically distinguishes, also, between the minor tranquillizers and the hypnotics and sedative-hypnotics. (The status of phenobarbitone, often considered to be an anti-anxiety drug, will be discussed below.)

Does the experimental evidence support clinical practice? We shall attempt to answer this question by focusing on a few of the anti-anxiety drugs that are widely used and on which there is reasonably extensive experimental data. These are meprobamate; chlordiazepoxide and the closely related diazepam; and phenobarbitone. What effects do these particular compounds have in common in various experimental situations, and by what behavioural or physiological mechanisms are they produced?

At the outset, it is most unlikely that the anti-anxiety drugs have a similar chemical action. Anti-anxiety drugs are found in four different chemical classes (Berger's classification[1]): the diphenyl methanes; the substituted amides (which includes the barbiturates); the propane diols (which includes meprobamate); and the benzodiazepines (which includes chlordiazepoxide and diazepam).

The clearest definition of the mode of action of the anti-anxiety drugs comes from experiments on behaviour. These experiments show unequivocally that chlordiazepoxide, meprobamate, and phenobarbitone have common properties that are qualitatively different from those of the phenothiazines or most of the barbiturates. On the other hand, the differences *among* these anti-anxiety drugs, while undoubtedly not without therapeutic significance, are largely quantitative: chlordiazepoxide and diazepam, for example, are much more potent than meprobamate and differ from meprobamate in the ratio between the doses producing different effects. The characteristic effects of the anti-anxiety drugs can be detected in various routine pharmacological screening procedures, but are defined more precisely by operant conditioning (lever pressing) methods.

PHARMACOLOGICAL SCREENING PROCEDURES

The " taming " of wild, aggressive animals by meprobamate, chlordiazepoxide, diazepam, and phenobarbitone has aroused considerable interest.[2, 3, 4] Following treatment with these drugs, ordinarily vicious monkeys can safely be petted or even poked although they are still " alert " and may show little impairment in moving about. " Taming " effects of a drug in these experiments can be distinguished from sedation by determining the drug's effects on aggressive behaviour relative to its depression of general activity or other routine behaviour.[3] In contrast to the anti-anxiety drugs, chlorpromazine or pentobarbitone do not "tame" because the animal is virtually immobile at the doses that appreciably attenuate aggressive behaviour.

Effects of the anti-anxiety drugs on " experimentally induced " aggressive behaviour resemble those obtained with " natural " aggressive behaviour.[5] Chlordiazepoxide and meprobamate are reported to selectively reduce or eliminate ferociousness in rats with septal lesions, " fighting " by pairs of mice placed on a charged grid, and fighting in mice previously isolated in individual cages.

The anti-convulsant and food intake tests are two other pharmacological situations in which the anti-anxiety drugs appear to have distinctive effects, according to Hanson and Stone[6]. These authors present data showing that meprobamate, chlordiazepoxide, and phenobarbitone " possess qualitatively similar types of anti-convulsant activity " in protecting mice against seizures induced by electroshock, pentylenetrazole, or strychnine. Hanson and Stone claim that the food-intake test " more clearly than any other, appears to be specific " for isolation of the anti-anxiety compounds. They show that non-sedative doses of meprobamate, chlordiazepoxide, and pentobarbitone all increase the amount of food eaten during 2-hr test periods by immature food-deprived rats. The phenothiazines or dexamphetamine, in contrast, decrease the amount eaten in the food-intake experiment.

Muscle relaxation at relatively low doses is another effect of meprobamate, chlordiazepoxide and phenobarbitone that has been observed in pharmacological screening. Muscle relaxant effects are measured in mice by noting the dose at which the animals fall off an inclined screen, and in cats by their " relaxed appearance " when suspended by the scruff of the neck.[7]

The pharmacological screening procedures show quite clearly that the anti-anxiety drugs do form a distinct class of compounds with a characteristic profile of action. They are all anti-convulsants and muscle relaxants, " tame " aggressive animals, and increase food intake, whereas compounds in the other drug classes act like the anti-anxiety drugs in at most three of the tests. Generalization of these empirical findings suggest that a new compound with a pharmacological screening profile similar to that of the anti-anxiety drugs would also prove to be an anti-anxiety drug when tested on humans.

The screening procedures sensitive to the action of the anti-anxiety drugs were determined empirically. They provide few clues as to what the mechanism (or mechanisms) of action of these drugs may be. It is hard to imagine a common behavioural or physiological mode of action that could account for the activity observed in such diverse situations as those just described. However, some recent operant conditioning studies provide some very plausible suggestions as to the fundamental action of the anti-anxiety drugs, as well as supporting the conclusion that these drugs comprise a distinct class.

OPERANT CONDITIONING PROCEDURES

The anti-anxiety drugs, the phenothiazines, and barbiturates are alike in depressing response rates in the continuous (Sidman) avoidance situation[8] in which the animal must repeatedly press a lever to prevent the occurrence of shock. Quantitative differences are observed, with the benzodiazepines especially having large differences between the minimum effective dose and the dose at which the animals fail to press the lever to turn off the shock.

The anti-anxiety drugs are rather inactive in the conventional " discrete trial " or " simultaneous " classical avoidance situation (see Fig. 1), in which possible shock is preceded by a 5-sec noise warning signal. The animal is shocked if it fails to press the lever during the warning. Meprobamate and chlordiazepoxide do not affect response below toxic doses,[4] whereas the

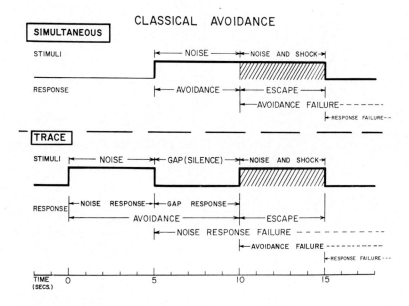

FIG. 1. Sequence of stimulus presentations in " simultaneous " and " trace " classical avoidance trials. From Heise and McConnell[9].

major tranquillizers selectively block the response to the warning at low doses, and the barbiturates (except for phenobarbitone) block all responding.

When the " simultaneous " avoidance situation just described is converted to " trace " avoidance (" successive compound avoidance " is a better term) by inserting a 5-sec silent " gap " between noise warning and shock (Fig. 1), qualitative differences appear between meprobamate, chlordiazepoxide and phenobarbitone, and chlorpromazine, as illustrated in Fig. 2. At appropriate doses of the anti-anxiety drugs, rats that failed to respond during the warning frequently responded during the gap; with chlorpromazine the animals almost never responded during the gap.[9] In accounting for these results, Cook and Kelleher[5] suggest that " . . . drugs such as meprobamate increase

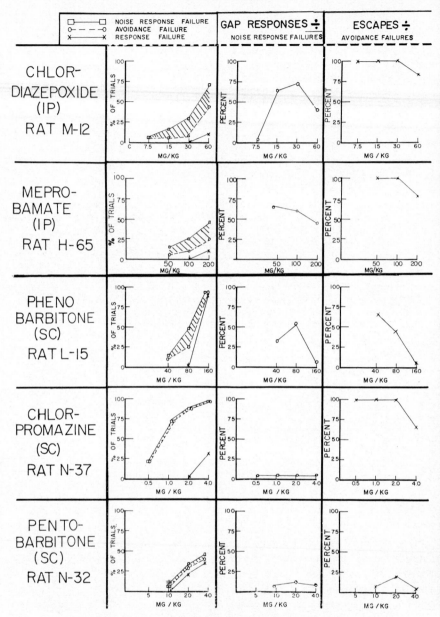

FIG. 2. Representative dose-response curves obtained with various drugs in
" trace " classical avoidance. The lined area shows " gap " responses, occurring
when the rat failed to respond during the initial noise but did not fail to avoid
(and did not receive a shock). The second column shows the conditional
probability of a gap response (gap responses/opportunities) and the third column
shows the conditional probability of an escape response (escape responses/
opportunities). Gap responses were high with chlordiazepoxide, meprobamate,
and phenobarbitone; escape responses were high with chlorpromazine; and
neither gap nor escape responses were often observed with pentobarbitone.
From Heise and McConnell[9].

the latency of conditioned avoidance responses, while chlorpromazine causes more complete block of all avoidance behaviour ". More recent work (unpublished) supports this interpretation.

Investigations of " response-contingent punishment ", more subjectively and less accurately described as " conflict ", make a significant step toward

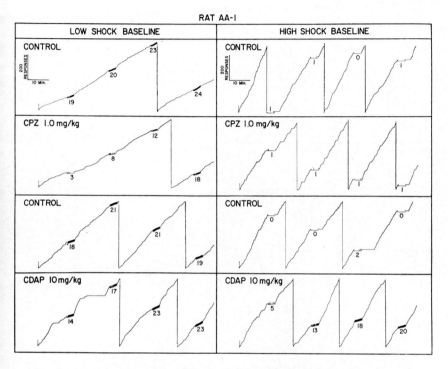

FIG. 3. Cumulative response records showing the effects of chlordiazepoxide (CDAP), and chlorpromazine (CPZ) on a " punishment discrimination ". Tone periods are indicated by the pen offsets; the responses that occurred during the tone periods, which were both rewarded with food and punished with shock, are indicated by upward strokes of the pen. Note that chlorpromazine *decreased* and chlordiazepoxide *increased* the number of responses made during the tone period. From Geller, Kulak, and Seifter[11].

precise specification of the behaviours affected by the anti-anxiety drugs. Geller[10, 11], investigated the effects of the anti-anxiety drugs on a " punishment discrimination ". Rats were trained to press a lever for milk delivered on the average once every 2 min (2-min VI). Then, at 15-min intervals, a tone was turned on for 3 min. During this tone or " conflict " period, every lever press was rewarded with milk (CRF), but was simultaneously punished by foot shock. Typical results are presented in Fig. 3.

Under control (non-drug) conditions, response during the tone period was suppressed and the animal received few shocks if the shock intensity was high. After administration of meprobamate, chlordiazepoxide, and phenobarbitone (measured against the " high shock " base-line), the rats responded much more frequently during the tone period and took many more shocks. Pentobarbitone and reserpine also had this effect. On the other hand, chlorpromazine, and other phenothiazines and dexamphetamine

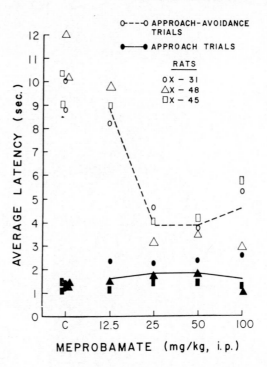

FIG. 4. Effects of meprobamate on average latency of responding to approach and approach-avoidance (" conflict ") tones for each of three rats. From Scheckel and McConnell[13].

(measured against the " low shock " base-line) actually intensified the suppression of lever pressing during the tone period. Differential effects between chlordiazepoxide and meprobamate, and chlorpromazine, have been reported for squirrel monkeys in a somewhat similar situation by Cook[12].

The distinctive action of the anti-anxiety drugs in countering the effects of response-contingent punishment is even more clearly demonstrated in a recent nicely-controlled experiment by Scheckel and McConnell[13]. Rats in a two-lever box were trained to obtain food pellets by pressing one lever on trials with a 2000 cps tone, and to press the other lever on trials with a

400 cps tone. Then shock was delivered following a small proportion (about 10 per cent) of the responses made on trials with the 400 cps tone, and training continued until responding became stable. Approach (2000 cps) and approach-avoidance (400 cps) trials were presented equally often, and in random order. Figures 4, 5, and 6 show that response latencies for control performance on the " approach-avoidance " trials were much longer than on the " approach " trials, and response failures were much more frequent. Figures 4 and 5 show that meprobamate and chlordiazepoxide shortened the latency of response on the approach-avoidance trials, but had little effect

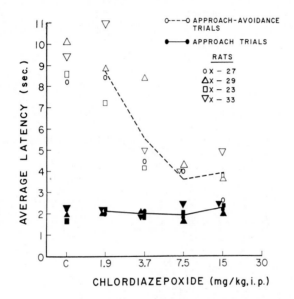

FIG. 5. Effects of chlordiazepoxide on response latency to approach and approach-avoidance tones. From Scheckel and McConnell[13].

on the latencies of the approach trials, which served as a concurrent control for non-specific stimulation or depression, depression of appetite, etc. Particular doses of these drugs also decreased the proportion of response failures on the approach-avoidance trials. Chlorpromazine (Fig. 6), on the other hand, neither decreased the latencies of the approach-avoidance trials nor decreased the proportion of response failures.

In analyzing their results, Scheckel and McConnell consider two principal ways in which meprobamate and chlordiazepoxide could increase the rat's tendency to perform the punished response in the approach-avoidance trials: the drugs could either enhance approach tendencies or attenuate the learned avoidance of the lever. They reject the former explanation because " stimulant " drugs like dexamphetamine do not increase response tendencies

on the approach-avoidance trials, and because meprobamate, chlordiazepoxide, and phenobarbitone increased response on the approach-avoidance
trials at doses that did not affect or even increased the latency on the
approach trials. Instead, the authors argue that the anti-anxiety drugs
attenuated " passive avoidance " behaviour—the learned tendency not to
press the lever as a consequence of punishment for lever pressing during

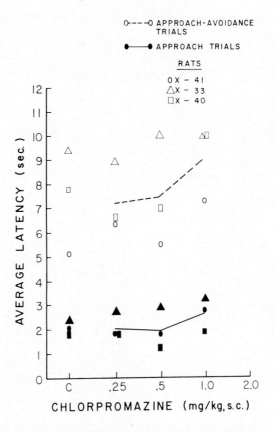

FIG. 6. Effects of chlorpromazine on response latency to approach and approach-
avoidance tones. From Scheckel and McConnell[13].

training. A similar explanation seems to apply to Geller's " punishment
discrimination " described above.

After surveying the effects of drugs in a large number of experiments
Scheckel and McConnell conclude that in passive avoidance experiments,
where the subject is punished if he *does* perform a particular response,
meprobamate and chlordiazepoxide increase the probability of that response
and chlorpromazine is inactive. In active avoidance such as the simultaneous

classical avoidance previously described, where the subject is punished if it does *not* perform a particular response, chlorpromazine decreases the probability of that response, and meprobamate and chlordiazepoxide are quite inactive.

The hypothesis that the anti-anxiety drugs attenuate responses suppressed by punishment or, more specifically, passive avoidance behaviour, has been extended by Scheckel and McConnell to account for increases produced by these drugs in the rate of responding on certain schedules of positively reinforced behaviour, as reported by Cook[12], Kelleher, Fry, Deegan and Cook et al.[14], and others. Chlordiazepoxide and meprobamate increase response rates on FI (fixed interval) and DRL (differential reinforcement of low rates) and other schedules in which response rate is slow or characterized by pauses, while chlorpromazine decreases the rate. An example of this " stimulation " of fixed interval performance is the monkey shown in Fig. 7. Scheckel and McConnell point to evidence that responses made during certain portions of these schedules (e.g. immediately following a reinforcement) may have aversive properties since they are never reinforced, and passive avoidance behaviour, indicated by " pausing ", may develop. Hence attenuation of passive avoidance behaviour by anti-anxiety drugs may shorten or eliminate pausing, and thus increase over-all rate.

The operant conditioning experiments support the conclusions derived from the pharmacological tests: that chlordiazepoxide (and diazepam), meprobamate, and phenobarbitone usually produce similar effects in a particular test—effects which are often qualitatively different from those of the phenothiazines or other barbiturates. The class of anti-anxiety drugs thus defined must include phenobarbitone, even though it is a hypnotic at high doses and a barbiturate, because in most respects it has the same type of actions as the other anti-anxiety drugs.

Most of the tests selected to bring out distinctive effects of the anti-anxiety drugs were far too complex to permit accurate identification of the types of behaviour affected by the anti-anxiety drugs. That is why the experiments showing that the anti-anxiety drugs attenuate the suppression of behaviour by response-contingent punishment, i.e. " conflict ", are so provocative: here is behaviour that is well-defined, that is affected quite differently by the anti-anxiety drugs than by other classes of drugs, and appears to have considerable generality.

The type of behaviour affected by the anti-anxiety drugs is defined still more precisely if one accepts Scheckel and McConnell's contention that these drugs attenuate passive avoidance. Solomon[15] has pointed to the ubiquity of passive avoidance, on both the animal and human level. Passive avoidance—learning *not* to do something—is the most probable response to punishment. One might speculate that, in addition to the usual repertoire of appropriate passive avoidance responses, the anxious person has learned

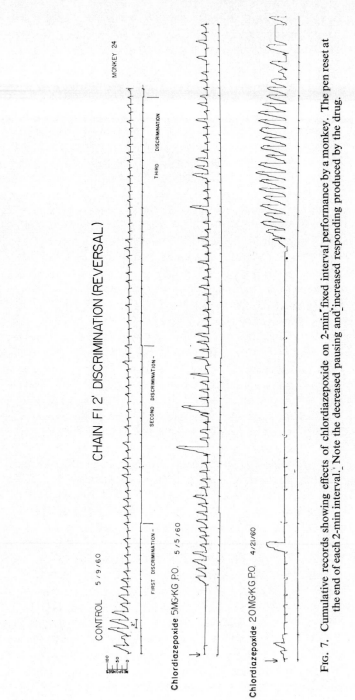

FIG. 7. Cumulative records showing effects of chlordiazepoxide on 2-min fixed interval performance by a monkey. The pen reset at the end of each 2-min interval. Note the decreased pausing and increased responding produced by the drug.

many *inappropriate* passive avoidance responses in his attempts to cope with real and imaginary dangers and conflicts. Under these circumstances, drugs which attenuate these passive avoidance responses might well be beneficial.

ELECTROPHYSIOLOGICAL STUDIES

An authoritative review[16] of the evidence on the site of action of central nervous system depressants stated in 1961, " We are still quite ignorant of the precise neural mechanisms of the action of any drug affecting the central nervous system ". This assertion is, of course, still true today. Nevertheless, some general conclusions concerning the central nervous system effects of the anti-anxiety drugs can be drawn—conclusions that are generally consistent with those based on behaviour.

Following Domino[16], a " profile " can be established for each drug based on its effects on the cortex, thalamus, hypothalamus, limbic system, brain stem reticular formation, and spinal cord. As predicted from their behavioural effects, the profiles for meprobamate and chlordiazepoxide are essentially similar, and quite different from those of pentobarbitone and phenobarbitone, or chlorpromazine. Relatively light doses of meprobamate and chlordiazepoxide depress principally (though not exclusively) the thalamus, limbic system, and spinal reflexes, especially polysynaptic reflexes. Perhaps most suggestive is Schallek, Zabransky and Kühn's[17] demonstration that chlordiazepoxide raised the threshold for inducing afterdischarge in the limbic system; similar effects were obtained with meprobamate by Kletzkin and Berger[18]. The " calming " of ferocious " septal " rats by meprobamate and chlordiazepoxide, cited earlier, is, of course, consistent with these observations. The depression of the limbic system by the anti-anxiety drugs—the amygdala is apparently particularly affected—is also not incompatible with the hypothesis that these drugs attenuate passive avoidance.

Chlorpromazine and the barbiturates have distinctly different profiles from meprobamate and chlordiazepoxide.[16] According to Schallek *et al.*[17], chlorpromazine does not depress and may even stimulate the thalamus and amygdala. Both phenobarbitone and pentobarbitone, on the other hand, generally depress all sites included in the profile.[16] Although phenobarbitone was placed in the same class as meprobamate and chlordiazepoxide on the basis of its effects on behaviour, it clearly must be classified quite separately from meprobamate and chlordiazepoxide on the basis of its effects on the central nervous system.

REFERENCES

1. BERGER, J. M., In *Drugs and Behavior*, Eds. Uhr, L. M. and Miller, J. G., Wiley, New York, 1960
2. HENDLEY, C. D., LYNES, T. E. and BERGER, F. M., *Fed. Proc.* **15**, 436 (1954).

3. HEISE, G. A. and BOFF, E., *Fed. Proc.* **20**, 393 (1961).
4. RANDALL, L. O., HEISE, G. A., SCHALLEK, W., BAGDON, R. E., BANZIGER, R., BORIS, A., MOE, R. A. and ABRAMS, W. B., *Curr. ther. Res.* **3**, 405 (1961).
5. COOK, L. and KELLEHER, R. T., *Ann. Rev. Pharmacol.* **3**, 205 (1963).
6. HANSON, H. and STONE, C. A., In *Animal and Clinical Pharmacologic Techniques in Drug Evaluation*, Eds. Nodine, J. H. and Siegler, P. E., Yearbook Medical Publishers, Chicago, 1964.
7. RANDALL, L. O., SCHALLEK, W., HEISE, G. A., KEITH, E. F. and BAGDON, R. E., *J. Pharmacol. exp. Ther.* **129**, 163 (1960).
8. HEISE, G. A. and BOFF, E., *Psychopharmacologia (Berl.)* **3**, 264 (1962).
9. HEISE, G. A. and MCCONNELL, H., In *Proceedings of the Third World Congress of Psychiatry* II, Ed. CLEGHORN, R. A., University of Toronto Press, Toronto, 1961.
10. GELLER, I., In *Psychomatic Medicine*, Eds. Nodine, J. H. and Moyer, J. H., Lea and Febiger, Philadelphia, 1962.
11. GELLER, I., KULAK, J. T. and SEIFTER, J., *Psychopharmacologia (Berl.)* **3**, 374 (1962).
12. COOK, L., In *Animal Behavior and Drug Action*, Eds. Steinberg, H., De Reuck, A. V. S. and Knight, J., Churchill, London, 1964.
13. SCHECKEL, C. and MCCONNELL, H., to be published.
14. KELLEHER, R. T., FRY, W., DEEGAN, J. and COOK, L., *J. Pharmacol. exp. Ther.* **133**, 271 (1961).
15. SOLOMON, R. L., *Amer. Psychologist* **19**, 239 (1964).
16. DOMINO, E. F., *Ann. Rev. Pharmacol.* **2**, 215 (1962).
17. SCHALLEK, W., ZABRANSKY, F. and KÜHN, A., *Arch. int. Pharmacodyn.* **149**, 467 (1964).
18. KLETZKIN, M. and BERGER, F. M., *Proc. Soc. exp. Biol. (N.Y.)* **100**, 681 (1959).

DISCUSSION

OPENER: MAURICE PARTRIDGE:

I should like to thank Dr. Linford Rees and his co-organizers for the invitation to this very interesting symposium. I feel less happy about the request that I should address you, for I have no message other than a few pedestrian thoughts arising from what you may well regard as rather casual clinical observations. But if one is going to speak on anxiety and drugs, I suppose one should address oneself to the question: What are the drugs to use if any? For we have recently been warned, at another conference elsewhere, against drugs in general as being " ego-dissolvers ". Be that as it may (and it must presumably be better to do without them if one can), if one must use some, what an array there has been. Who now remembers the carbon dioxide treatment; or mephenesin; or its more elaborate cousin " Anxine "; or the polypharmaceutical product " Sedaltin "; or benactyzine? Who now uses methylpentynol? Perhaps many, but I do not know them. It seems to me that the drugs now most popularly prescribed for the treatment of anxiety—and here I am not at all at variance with Dr. Jenner— and therefore most deserving of consideration, are (1) what one may loosely call the tranquillizers, subdivided into (a) meprobamate, (b) the phenothiazines, and (c) chlordiazepoxide, and its relative diazepam, and (2) the barbiturates.

Of these, first meprobamate. It is possible, as often, to pick perplexing discrepancies from the literature. For example, Heller's study[1] found the results unimpressive. Uhlenhuth and his co-workers, mentioned by Dr. Jenner, found it effective if prescribed by one doctor but not if prescribed by the other, though the trial was double blind. Raymond and his collaborators,[3] in a double-blind trial at St. George's, found that it conferred no benefit at all. If, in face of such conflict, one has to form one's own view, my personal old-fashioned clinical impression is that this substance is expensive, unreliable and unsatisfactory. Where it does exert an effect, this is so often, though not always, in the direction of making the patient feel mildly drunk, which some like and some do not, and the patient who likes that effect in one setting may not like it in another. It is certainly an addictive substance. I have long ceased to use it.

Next, the phenothiazines, and taking chlorpromazine as the prototype. Rees and Lambert[4] in a large series of patients taking very small doses over a very short period of time found that chlorpromazine exerted an appreciable effect. Merry and his associates[5] with a small series of cases with much larger doses and over a longer period of time found its effect negligible. Raymond[3] in the study previously referred to, with a moderately large series of cases on moderate doses over the same period as Rees and Lambert, found it quite ineffective. As often, one wonders where one is. My own impression, and it is no more than that, is that, although the phenothiazines can be most effective in treating psychotic agitation or anxiety, such as may form an integral part of involutional melancholia and of some cases of manic-depressive psychosis and schizophrenia, they confer no appreciable benefit on cases with neurotic anxiety. Dr. Denham told us yesterday that he found perphenazine (as opposed to chlorpromazine) useful in anxiety, but that does not accord with my personal experience.

This brings us to chlordiazepoxide. Contradictions in the literature here are that Jenner et al.[6] found this superior to a placebo in a controlled trial, and that the patients preferred it to amylobarbitone. They are supported to some extent by Gore and McComisky[7] who found both chlordiazepoxide and amylobarbitone superior to a placebo, and who themselves thought the effects of chlordiazepoxide superior to those of amylobarbitone, though their patients did not. On the other hand, Schwarzberg and Van de Castle[8], matching chlordiazepoxide and meprobamate against a placebo, found chlordiazepoxide the least effective of the three. If, again, one has to make up one's own mind, my feeling, from a limited and unscientific experience and despite the opinions of the St. Thomas's school, is that chlordiazepoxide is almost an inert substance if given in ordinary doses to anyone except the elderly. Its striking capsule makes it look as though it is going to do something to you, and so may on occasion and with luck have a suggestive effect. This, together with the fact that it seems harmless (and a case has been reported of spontaneous recovery after taking 1630 mg in an alleged suicidal attempt)—and despite the fact that Dr. Dally has reported it to be addictive—has caused me still to prescribe it from time to time in those cases where my weakness of will is such that I feel I must prescribe something, and where I fear that the patient may develop a dependence upon barbiturates. Apart from that, I am not quite sure that it may not have some very limited use in those cases where the injudicious intake of alcohol constitutes a threat to the well-being of the only partially co-operative patient. This is only a tentative thought, arising from very few cases, but I am not sure that chlordiazepoxide may not be an agent which can tide a person along so that he does not start to drink too early in the day, and which can help the partially co-operative patient to keep his intake of alcohol within bounds. This very limited and dubious possible use remains to be tested further for what it is worth. Of chlordiazepoxide's newly arrived cousin diazepam, I can say nothing because I have not yet used it. Conversation with my clinician colleagues does not particularly encourage me to do so.

Otherwise, as an old-fashioned clinician dependent on his impressions, I come down squarely, as an old square should, on the side of the barbiturates, if drugs are really necessary in the treatment of neurotic anxiety, using them in the pious hope that they are only an ancillary part of the treatment, and watching their use with care as regards dosage and the possible development of dependence, which last, I think, is not likely to occur so long as the dose— even over a period of many weeks—is kept to less than 12 grains over each period of 24 hr.

REFERENCES

1. HELLER, G. C., WALTON, D. and BLACK, D. A., *J. ment. Sci.* **103**, 581 (1957).
2. UHLENHUTH, E. H., CANTER, A., NEUSTADT, J. O. and PAYSON, H. E., *Amer. J. Psychiat.* **115**, 905 (1959).
3. RAYMOND, M. J., LUCAS, C. J., BEESLEY, M. L. and O'CONNELL, B. A., *Brit. med. J.* **ii**, 63 (1957).
4. REES, W. L. and LAMBERT, C., *J. ment. Sci.* **101**, 834 (1955).
5. MERRY, J., PARGITER, R. A. and MUNRO, H., *Amer. J. Psychiat.* **113**, 988 (1957).
6. JENNER, F. A. and KERRY, R. J., *J. ment. Sci.* **107**, 583 (1961).
7. GORE, C. P. and McCOMISKY, J. G., In *Proceedings of the Third World Congress of Psychiatry* II, Ed. Cleghorn, R. A., University of Toronto Press, Toronto, 1961.
8. SCHWARTZBERG, A. Z. and VAN DE CASTLE, R. W., *Amer. J. Psychiat.* **117**, 922 (1961).

OPENER: E. BERESFORD DAVIES:

Almost everybody knows what anxiety is, because he can feel it himself and recognize it in others. At the same time the feeling defies definition. We are forced therefore to describe it in indirect terms mainly by its effects, which makes it very difficult even for an expert to be sure that the meaning he gives to the word will be correctly understood by his colleagues; so it is not surprising that the general medical mind is confused about anxiety.

For example, anxiety is said to be a component of many depressive states: so much so that they have on occasion been called anxiety neuroses.[1] This is an interesting reversal of the trend of a decade and a half ago when, possibly as a result of a reaction to war-time anxiety, this diagnosis went out of fashion and there was a move to regard all cases presenting with anxiety as conditions of concealed depression.

Again, the word anxiety may be used to form part of newer, longer words such as anxiety-depersonalization neurosis[2] which describe conditions that we recognize as old friends with new titles originally described by workers whose ideas are no longer fashionable (Freud). Or again less high-sounding names but with the superficial attraction of alliteration are used, such as " housebound housewives ". This term disguises the well-known condition of widespread phobia which paralyses its victims.

We may not be in quite the same semantic muddle in relation to anxiety as we are to depression but there is certainly confusion, as is shown by what happened with one general practitioner of whom I know. The doctor wanted the husband of a " housebound housewife " to be seen by a marriage guidance counsellor on account of his supposed cruelty to his wife, who was chained to her sink, by his neglect of a share of the housework.

We cannot judge, owing to our ignorance of the pathological basis of anxiety, whether there is such a specific illness as anxiety-neurosis in the sense that there is an illness like lobar pneumonia and we must therefore be ever careful to separate hypothesis from experiment when we are conducting trials of drugs. In fact there is something to be said for adopting a cookery book method of investigation by which one records the signs and symptoms of an illness on the one hand, and its means of treatment on the other, as the ingredients of a particular dish and its preparation respectively. The results can then be surveyed pragmatically and subjected to statistical analysis. However, if we use this method we must also be sure that in describing our experiments we do not naively use terms which are already loaded with prejudice, or unconsciously associated with one another without rational basis.

The disorder in which anxiety is most prominent, with the least admixture of symptoms and signs of some other disease process, is the classical severe state of anxiety described abundantly in the literature generally and by workers of the Freudian school, who call the basic affect *angst*, which is not adequately translated by the English word anxiety. This state is variously called acute anxiety, panic attack or phobic state, and is characterized by intolerable anxiety, sometimes without any immediate cognitive connection but rather more often attaching to an idea in the form of a phobia of some kind. Most of the physiological accompaniments of fear are present and the attack usually subsides only when the patient succeeds in escaping from his immediate environment, whether this be internal, that is in his own mind, or in the outer world.

This kind of illness appears to be the purest form of anxiety and one is struck by its apparently psychological nature despite its physical concomitants.

This can be contrasted with the state of affairs in endogenous depression where the anxiety, if this indeed is the name we should give to this part of the affect in that condition, is closely associated with other symptoms and signs which may be psychological, such as depression and self-criticism, or physical such as restlessness and sleeplessness.

I think this state in endogenous depression is qualitatively different from *angst* and that it is better described either in psychological terms such as loss of confidence or courage, and absence of the power of concentration and decision, or in physical terms such restlessness or agitation, with repetitive useless behaviour. This is not to deny that in milder or early cases of the disease anxiety may arise in the patient from his awareness of his failing powers, just as in early schizophrenia anxiety and depression acting together may cause a suicidal attempt while the patient has still enough grasp to realize that he is in a desperate state. Thus, in depressive illness we may see secondary feelings of apprehension more akin to worry or concern than fear.

I therefore think it very important to distinguish between these two pathological states, not least to avoid bringing discredit on valuable remedies. It is well known—any practising psychiatrist can find it out for himself—that successful treatment with an effective antidepressant drug given to a patient who is suffering from endogenous depression has the result of reducing apprehension, concern and tension, at the same time as there is relief of the depressive signs and symptoms themselves.

We can contrast this with the problems of treatment of the phobic states. I have already mentioned the much more psychological aspect of the state of these patients with severe anxiety, and their characteristic concentration on the self, with acute awareness of their feelings despite the accompanying lack of insight which they almost always display. It is characteristic that these patients try to deal with their anxiety by psychological mechanisms such as the production of phobias or the manipulation of themselves in relation to the environment. I think we all have to admit that so far no drug has been found which has a direct or decisive effect on these severe states of anxiety unless it is given in doses which are so large as to produce paralysis of the higher centres of the nervous system.

Treatment has to be in part psychological, and whatever means is adopted, whether psychotherapy in the formal sense or the newer fashionable treatment by desensitization, the method is the same, namely to produce an alteration in the manner in which the patient attaches emotion to his immediate state of being.

Clearly we must agree, unless we are prepared to take a dualist standpoint, that the anxiety must be subserved somewhere at a neurophysiological level. Such success as may be obtained in treatment, however, suggests the disease is more related to faulty patterns of behaviour than to pathological neurophysiological processes—a contrast to what seemingly happens in endogenous depression, where the basic pathological state is likely to be a neurochemical fault.

Naturally we have to ask whether there may be a disease process which primarily affects the mechanism whereby anxiety is produced. Obviously if this were the case then the psychological aspects of anxiety which loom so large clinically would have to be seen as concomitant secondary signs and symptoms, like the thunder which accompanies lightning, while treatment would have to be directed to the underlying pathology of the anxiety-producing mechanism. Here no doubt drug therapy would have great scope, as we know that it has in the analogous disease of endogenous depression.

I have now taken two very clear-cut conditions. If only depression were always obviously endogenous, and anxiety were always obviously phobic, then our problems would be a great deal easier. However, this is not always the case. We are confronted by all kinds of admixtures of conditions. It is not at all uncommon to see a patient with reactive depressive problems, some degree of true endogenous depression, as well as lifelong tendency to anxiety under stress. Confusion becomes worse confounded when in a trial of drugs such patients are grouped together without adequate analysis: the results are then incomprehensible to other psychiatrists working on what they think are the same problems. No wonder we get widely divergent results in clinical trials, and we are divided at best by misunderstanding and at worst by prejudice.

One must also stress the constant difficulty of treating phobic patients with psychotropic drugs because of the readiness with which these patients produce psychological reactions during the course of treatment. The sources of confusion are first an improvement or deterioration in the patient's condition due to an internal event in the patient's mind not connected with the drug; second, an external event to which he has made a response again unconnected with the drug. If the therapist, in trying to make his treatment as scientific as possible, deliberately creates a detached attitude—in other words if he does not load the psychotropic substances he is about to give with therapeutic value and expectations—he is not likely to get good results. It does not matter whether he knows what he is giving, or does not know as in a double-blind trial. His results, particularly in the treatment of states of severe anxiety, are likely to be dominated by factors in the experimental situation which have nothing whatsoever to do with the pharmacological properties of the substances he is using. I am stressing this, not because I have a remedy for this difficult situation, but because failure to recognize this truth leads to some extraordinary findings from clinical trials whether positive or negative.

REFERENCES

1. MAYER-GROSS, W., SLATER, E. and ROTH, M., *Clinical Psychiatry*, 2nd ed., Cassell, London (1960). (Quoting West and Dally.)
2. ROTH, M., *Proc. roy. Soc. Med.* **52**, 587 (1959).

GENERAL DISCUSSION

CHAIRMAN: I want to make use of the Chairman's prerogative of saying a few words about the problems of the anxiety states at the beginning of the discussion and, particularly, to give you some of the views from St. Thomas's.

We have an annual new and old attendance rate of 17,000 and using the Barcroft-blood flow method we have had difficulty in finding 20 patients recently among these who seem to be suffering from true anxiety states.

On the other hand we have a wide variety of depressive states stretching from those simulating anxiety states to the classical endogenous depressions. Dr. Birley[1] while working in my department studied the further history of 200 patients in whom I had advised leucotomy for long continued (5–6 years) tension states. A surprising number of these patients developed typical depressive episodes subsequently. Examination of the case records in retrospect showed that adequate antidepressant therapy had not been given to these patients prior to the decision to undertake leucotomy. At the present time patients who are referred to us with tension states for an opinion about leucotomy are all treated with continuous sleep, a combination of iproniazid and amitriptyline in full doses, and a course of ECT. Over the last 6 months few cases have had to be referred for leucotomy. It is obvious that we were previously treating as tension states by leucotomy, cases which we have now shown can be adequately controlled by antidepressant drugs and ECT. Many of these patients had been ill with apparent tension states for up to eight years or more.

These " tension " states must now be regarded as masked depressions, and often present as cases of chronic anxiety states in a previously good personality. Cases of anxiety state with a previous good personality are often treated unsuccessfully with chlordiazepoxide. We regard the treatment of these cases as the same as atypical depression, and we now treat all such patients with phenelzine, isocarboxazid or iproniazid with or without chlordiazepoxide. The MAOI is the most important one for relief of the symptoms

The next group that I would like to consider are the mixed ones, with the fatigue syndrome characteristic of atypical depression occurring together with the usual features of endogenous depression. Such cases do very well with both groups of drugs given together.

The last group are the endogenous depressions. Even these may present with anxiety symptoms. Such patients should be treated with ECT and the antidepressant drugs and in particular, amitriptyline. Amitriptyline is itself a sedative drug as well as an antidepressant and, in fact, in patients who do not sleep well at night I give amitriptyline 75 to 100 mg at night and up to 50 mg during the day.

Although this Symposium is entitled " The Scientific Basis ", I think it is important that we appreciate the part played by good clinical observation in the assessment of therapy. Double-blind controlled trials and statistics can be used to confirm observations that have been made at the bedside but are no substitute for them.

RUSSELL BARTON (*Colchester*): Our subject has been the scientific basis of drug treatment in psychiatry.

Although the papers have been interesting and, I accept, have great intrinsic merit, not much of what has been said has been germane to our subject.

By science (and implied is a positive science as opposed to a normative one), I understand a systematized collection of facts obtained by observation—coincidental and repeated observations—hypothesis and experiment.

Hypothesis is a supposition which connects facts in a regular manner. Experiment is a deliberate arrangement of facts and conditions of an hypothesis, so that the consequence can be tested by direct observation.

Psychiatry is the science of abnormalities of experience and behaviour.

In spite of the problems occasioned by subjective experience, it cannot be rejected. The psychologist cannot follow Watson and other behaviourists, unless he wants to divorce himself from psychiatry. I won't go into these problems here because they are discussed in my paper which was published in the *Lancet*.[2]

Animal experiments do not provide a scientific basis for drug treatment in psychiatry, however interesting and useful in physiology; however attractive and plausible the speculations which arise they are not scientific.

The enthusiasms and prejudices for the effects of drugs aired by many of our speakers, including yourself, sir, are not scientific.

Yet clinical impressions are absolutely essential in treatment. Please do not let me be misunderstood, without this intuitive approach we could not treat anyone.

Much of the elegant super-structure we have heard described is based on foundations that are at best speculative and at worst fantasy.

HAROLD PALMER (*St. Albans*): I very much appreciated Dr. Beresford Davies' remarks about failures in anxiety. I have never yet encountered a case which I, personally, would have labelled anxiety state as opposed to masked depression who did not at some time experience a phobia. During the war time we saw a tremendous number of anxiety states and I believe they were real anxiety states with no evidence of masked depression. They were afraid—of the blitz, of bombs, in fact of being killed. To some extent they were phobic, they were dominated by this, and I feel that Dr. Beresford Davies' point is sustained. I would suggest that the anxiety state is a general manifestation of a focal phobia, in the same way that a septicaemia is a general spread of a local abscess. In more typical depressives and, of course, in schizophrenia one does not find these phobic situations. The unarguable residue of the anxiety state as I first described it and as we met it with our soldiers, is the phobia. If this is indeed true then we may ask " Have we got a drug that attacks the phobic situation? ". In my experience the answer is definitely " No ".

CHAIRMAN: I think that we should congratulate Dr. Palmer on these observations and at the same time acknowledge the fact that many of our present treatment methods in psychiatry such as ether abreaction and continuous sleep are based on his earlier work.

J. D. POLLITT (*London*): I would like to support Dr. Palmer in his view. Many of these so-called anxiety cases are masked depressions. I believe strongly that anxiety states in young people are really a manifestation of endogenous depression. Over the past four years I have been examining the cases that respond to the monoamine oxidase inhibitors and have found that there is some evidence of a physiological shift in sleep, diurnal rhythm, libido, appetite, weight in some degree which do not occur in true anxiety states.

P. H. ROGERS (*Northampton*): In relation to what Dr. Pollitt has just said, I would like to mention an impression, that episodes in children in which anxiety has been dominant have apparently often been precipitated by one of the viral infections of childhood. These may be the strict analogue of the post viral depressive illnesses of adult life.

DEREK RICHTER: May I bring up a conflict of views. Dr. Himwich has taken the view that drug therapy can do something to the underlying disease process whatever that is, whereas on the other hand Dr. Denham and others regard drugs as simply correcting symptoms. In any case psychotherapy is generally given as an adjunct to drug treatment: is this any more or any less effective than the drugs in dealing either with the underlying disease or with symptoms?

CHAIRMAN: I am convinced that this conflict is a red herring. What is important from the practical point of view is that the drugs work. When quinine was brought in, I would remind you that this was an empiric remedy and it was Sydenham who said " Stop all this damn theorizing, this stuff works ". It took over 250 years to invent a microscope to show why.

BERESFORD DAVIES: Dr. Richter has raised an important point about the part played by psychotherapy. When drugs are used, the manner in which they are given, the personality of the doctor and the expectations which are aroused by their use may be the decisive factors in what happens to the patient.

CHAIRMAN: What worries me about this idea about one's personality being the therapeutic factor is how the patients know that they are going to get better on the seventh to tenth day. How do they also know that if you stop the drug, they are not going to relapse until seven days after. This cannot be due to suggestion and this is why I don't agree about the value of suggestion.

HAROLD PALMER (*St. Albans*): We all know that dreaming increases in anxiety states and the type of dream may alter. Some work we are undertaking suggests that drugs affect dreaming. It is now possible to quantitate some aspects of dreaming and I wonder if this could be used with advantage in studies on drug action.

F. STEEL (*London*): I should like to make a few clinical observations. I have found chlordiazepoxide effective in obsessional anxiety; meprobamate very good for autonomic anxiety. With regard to this question of antidepressant drugs, I am convinced that it is immaterial who gives them. It is the drug and not the person who prescribes them that matters. Two observations are relevant. First a general practitioner may try several drugs ineffectively before hitting on a specific antidepressant which then has a miraculous result. Secondly, prior to the advent of the antidepressant drugs psychiatrists tried many medicaments, but none worked. Now we get results with antidepressants, yet our personalities remain the same!

CHAIRMAN: Before we close the discussion, although it is not strictly relevant to this session, I should like to take the Chairman's prerogative of raising the question of phenothiazine basal ganglia damage. This has been mentioned in the medical press recently and subsequently exaggerated out of all proportion in the national press.

In fact such cases are extraordinarily rare, and even so, virtually confined to patients with previous brain damage.

The national press has done great disservice to patients and I should like to go on record as stating that this rare effect should not be regarded as a bar to the use of phenothiazines.

F. STEEL (*London*): I quite agree.

REFERENCES

1. BIRLEY, J. L. T., *Brit. J. Psychiat.* **110**, 211 (1964).
2. BARTON, R., *Lancet* **ii**, 566 (1963).

SESSION V
GENERAL CONSIDERATIONS
Chairman: WILLIAM SARGANT

INTERACTIONS INVOLVING DRUGS USED IN PSYCHIATRY

JOHN MARKS

Summary—The place of any therapy depends on the relationship between the effectiveness of the treatment, the incidence and severity of the side effects and the mortality and morbidity of the disease. The responsibility for selection of treatment for the individual patient must always remain ultimately with the physician, fully aware of the relevant facts. The therapeutic value of such combined therapy has been stated previously in the Symposium.

The problem that has been outlined is the complexity of the interactions of the centrally-acting drugs which the physician may wish to use with other drugs and with ingredients in the food. While pharmacologists have the responsibility for checking for such interactions in the direction of known or suspected areas, progress in unsuspected areas of interaction can only occur with good observation and reliable reporting by the clinician.

Résumé—La place de toute thérapie dépend de la relation entre l'efficacité du traitement, la fréquence et la gravité des effets secondaires, le taux de mortalité et de morbidité de la maladie. La responsabilité pour le choix du traitement doit toujours incomber en fin de compte à chaque praticien pleinement conscient des faits présents.

Le problème qui a été souligné est la complexité de l'interaction des préparations ayant une action centrale qu'il peut souhaiter utiliser avec d'autres médicaments et avec d'autres ingrédients dans la nourriture. Tandis que les firmes pharmaceutiques ont la responsabilité de vérifier de telles interactions dans les zones connues ou suspectes, les progrès dans les zones d'interaction exemptes de soupçon ne peuvent être réalisés que grâce à une bonne observation et aux rapports sûrs du clinicien.

Zusammenfassung—Die Bedeutung, die einer Behandlungsform zukommt, wird bestimmt durch das Verhältnis, in dem Wirksamkeit, Häufigkeit und Schweregrad der Nebenerscheinungen sowie Mortalitäts—und Morbiditätsquote der betreffenden Krankheit zueinander stehen. Die Verantwortung für die Wahl einer bestimmten Behandlungsform muss letztlich immer in den Händen des einzelnen Arztes bleiben, der diese Wahl in voller Kenntnis der ausschlaggebenden Faktoren trifft.

Es wurde das Problem der komplexen Wechselwirkungen zwischen einem im ZNS angreifenden Medikament und anderen Medikamenten oder Nahrungsbestandteilen erörtert. Aufgabe der Herstellerfirmen ist es, solche Wechselwirkungen soweit sie bekannt sind oder vermutet werden zu überprüfen; ein Fortschritt in der Kenntnis bisher unvorhersehbarer Wechselwirkungen kann nur durch die gute Beobachtung und zuverlässige Berichterstattung des Klinikers erreicht werden.

OVER the past decade many active drugs have become available to the psychiatrist, and we may anticipate that the next few years will see the introduction of many more.

The major part of psychiatric therapy is at present symptomatic and perhaps for this reason the simultaneous use of two or more drugs is probably more common in this than in any other single speciality (Table 1).

In assessing the merits of any therapy it is essential to assess the risks involved in relation to the clinical therapeutic value. The efficacy of drug therapy, both single and combined, has been considered by others in this symposium. It must, however, be remembered that most active drugs and indeed even placebos have side effects. In the simultaneous use of several active drugs it is important to realize that not only may the desired activities summate or potentiate but interactions may take place between the side

TABLE 1. Combined Use of Drugs used in Psychiatry Expressed as Percentages of Prescriptions.[1]

Combined with	Chlorpromazine	Diazepines	Imipramine	MAOI's
Thymoleptics	4·8	7·0	2·0	4·3
MAOI's	2·2	6·6	5·3	—
Diazepines	2·5	—	8·9	16·7
Sedatives	25·5	13·3	8·1	6·4
Phenothiazines	1·6	4·8	18·0	15·2
Others	16·4	2·0	6·6	10·0
Nil	47·0	66·3	51·1	47·4

effects. It is equally important to realize that the majority of psychiatric patients who receive drug therapy come into the age group in which chronic physical disorders are common. Thus interactions can take place with therapy not under control of the psychiatrist (e.g. administered by an anaesthetist).

The consensus of opinion at the meeting and the figures based on actual dosage seems to favour combined therapy in certain patients. Nevertheless, it is important to appreciate the problems and these will be discussed here.

Following the lead of the title of the symposium, these results are considered from the viewpoint of the mode of interactions rather than by giving a mere catalogue. This should give general principles which could be applied to future compounds. Strictly speaking these reactions should be described as " undesirable effects " but the term " side effects " is now used in this context by accepted medical usage.

Drugs can produce side effects by interactions by the following mechanisms.

(1) Simple summation of side effects or summation of the main effects of one drug with the side effect of another.

(2) Interactions in which the specific action of the compound exposes an unusual side effect.

(3) Interactions in which an indirect action of the compound exposes an unusual side effect.

(1) *Simple Summation of Effects*

This is undoubtedly the most common type of interaction. It may involve summation of the side effects of the two drugs or potentiation of the main effect of one drug by the side effect of the other. Some of these summations which can be demonstrated readily in animals have not yet been described in humans. This difference is, however, probably related to dosage differences rather than species differences and it would appear probable that human reactions of the type may be expected.

It must be stressed that even in those cases in which the human reaction has been found, the incidence is usually extremely low. Some of the main categories of such summations are:

(a) Summation of central depressant effect
  e.g. (i) Phenothiazines and pethidine.[2-6] This may even reach the stage of producing death.
       (ii) Tranquillizers and sedatives with alcohol. Numerous reports of animal experiments and clinical deaths from such combination are to be found in the literature.[7-10]

(b) Summation of extrapyramidal effects
  e.g. Phenothiazines and reserpine producing parkinsonism.[11]

(c) Summation of parasympathetic effects
  e.g. Paralytic ileus due to amitriptyline and chlorpromazine.[12] This could also be a danger when a ganglion blocking drug is given with one of the parasympathomimetic psychotropic drugs.

(d) Potentiation of thyroid by thymoleptics
  e.g. Cardiac abnormality with imipramine and thyroxin.[13]

(e) Summation of hypotensive effects
  e.g. Phenothiazines can summate with most hypotensives.

(2) *Interactions in which the Specific Action of the Compound Exposes an Unusual Side Effect*

In the previous group individual side effects of each compound are clearly known and the anticipated summation takes place.

The second group differs from this in that the two compounds given individually do not show the side effect or show it only minimally. Given together, however, the potentiation of effect is so great that an unexpected side effect can occur.

The best example of this type of reaction is that of the hypertensive crises in patients taking monoamine oxidase inhibitors. Although these reactions were described for iproniazid in 1953[14] during its trial as an agent against tuberculosis, it is only within the past two years that these reactions have caused widespread interest. These hypertensive crises which can cause death by intracranial haemorrhage are similar to those associated with phaeochromocytoma. The mode of production of many of these reactions can now be explained but anomalies still exist.

Figure 1 gives a simplified account of catecholamine interactions. Under normal circumstances free catecholamines are rapidly broken down. During

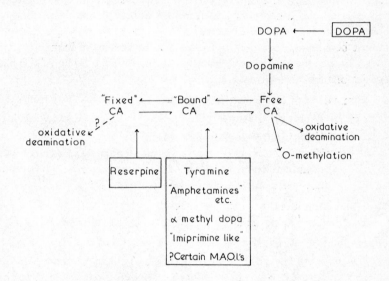

FIG. 1. Catecholamine interactions.

monoamine oxidase depletion, free or released catecholamines can stimulate receptors in the heart and blood vessels. Such a build up of active catecholamines at these receptor sites can occur by additional DOPA metabolism,[15-17] by their release from their *bound* form by various substances[18] or the release from the *fixed* form by reserpine.[19] This latter effect only gives receptor activation if the level of monoamine oxidase activity is too low to cause immediate breakdown. Such hypertensive crises in patients on monoamine oxidase inhibitors have been reported associated with:

(a) *The thymoleptics.* Imipramine and perhaps amitriptyline after monoamine oxidase inhibitors.[20-24] This is probably due to block of storage of free catecholamines.

(b) *Amphetamine-like substances.*[25-29] Probably mainly when given by injection. The mode of catecholamine release by these compounds has been described by Burn and Rand some years ago.[18]

(c) *Rauwolfia preparations.* In animals pretreatment with monoamine oxidase inhibitors alters the sedative effect of reserpine to stimulation,[30] and produces hypertension.[31] In patients untoward effects have also been reported during treatment with reserpine or tetrabenazine following treatment with monoamine oxidase inhibitors.[32-34] Curiously, however, these have been in the nature of agitated delirium rather than hypertensive crises.

(d) *Alpha methyldopa.* In animals, pretreatment with monoamine oxidase inhibitors causes the normally hypotensive compound α-methyldopa to become hypertensive[35] due to catecholamine release. No clinical reports of the reaction are available but this compound should be regarded as a potential danger.

TABLE 2. Tyramine Content of Various Foods.

		Percentages
Cheeses	Roquefort	0·04
	Emmenthal	0·02–0·06
	Cheddar	0·1–0·4
	Edam	0·2
	Camembert	0·0008–0·2
	Liederkrantz	1·6
	Stilton	0·04
Beer		0·0002–0·0004
Wine		0·0001–0·0002
Fruit and Vegetable	Banana	0·0007
	Tomato	0·0004
	Plum	0·0006
	Avocado	0·002
	Potato	0·0001
	Orange	0·001

Sources.[47-51]

(e) *Local anaesthetic agents.* Cocaine which blocks catecholamine uptake and which is often given locally with adrenaline is a potential danger. A case has been reported in which this may have been a contributory cause.[36]

(f) *Cheese.* Blackwell[37] was the first to describe the association between the ingestion of cheese several hours after the dose of a monoamine oxidase inhibitor and a hypertensive crisis. From Great Britain a total of 67 cases has been described in which a fairly certain correlation exists.[27, 29, 38-46]

This reaction has been shown to be due to the absorption of tyramine from the cheese. Cheeses vary in their tyramine content (Table 2) but, normally, this tyramine is broken down by monoamine oxidase in the intestinal wall. When the monoamine oxidase both there and in the body generally is inhibited, free tyramine can be absorbed and then may release catechol-

O

amnes.[49, 52, 53]   The ingested dose of tyramine to cause this reaction in the human is probably usually about 10–20 mg but may be as low as 6 mg.[50]   Clinical evidence, backed by animal experiments, suggests that attacks due to tranylcypromine are most likely to occur after an evening cheese meal when the blood level of tranylcypromine is low.   (Last dose normally given at mid-day.)

(g) *Marmite*[54, 55] *and Bovril.*[56]   They have been suggested as a rare cause.   Their mode of action is at present unknown.

(h) *Broad beans.*   One case due to eating whole broad beans has been described.   The reaction is due to the presence of about 0·25 per cent DOPA in the pods.[58]   The effective ingested dose of DOPA is probably about 25–50 mg.[15–17]

(k) *Alcohol.*   This has been implicated by several authors.[29, 59–61] Recent studies[50] show that beer contains tyramine at a concentration of about 1–2 mg per pint and wines up to 15 mg per bottle.   Variability of the levels was not studied sufficiently but it appears likely that blood pressure raising levels might be achieved prior to intoxication.   The reaction is often atypical and potentiation of alcohol by a different method cannot be excluded (p. 198).

It must be appreciated that the present evidence suggests that all monoamine oxidase inhibitors can show this reaction with appropriate " trigger " compounds.

Although much is now known of these reactions several points still require elucidation:

(i) In addition to those cases in which another compound has been implicated a further 115 patients showing hypertensive crises have been reported in the British literature over the past two years.[14, 29, 62–78] Many of these were reported before the association with dietary items was recognized and can probably be explained on this basis but a recent report[29] shows that in 30 per cent of patients the hypertensive crises cannot at present, be explained in this way.   The majority of such incidents occur on tranylcypromine.

Other dietary factors may be involved.   The normal diet contains about 4000 mg phenylalanine and 3000 mg tyrosine per day derived from both animal and vegetable proteins.   Phenylalanine can be converted into tyrosine and this readily converted to DOPA.   Since the toxic dose of DOPA in a patient on monoamine oxidase inhibitors is about 25–50 mg the rate of conversion does not need to be very great for a toxic level to be reached. Decarboxylation of tyrosine to tyramine normally requires bacterial action but this could, theoretically, occur in the alimentary canal.   Some decarboxylation can also take place in the kidney.   The toxic dose of tyramine with monoamine oxidase inhibitors is as low as 6 mg so that this is another possible cause of trouble. A three or greater fold rise in urinary excretion of tyramines in patients on monoamine oxidase inhibitors with levels up to 2·4 mg/day has indeed been reported.[79]

Tryptophan in the diet cannot be incriminated for although it has been shown to produce drowsiness, hyper-reflexia and ataxia after monoamine oxidase inhibitors[80, 81] hypertension is not seen although the dose used (7–15 g/day) is well above that derived from the diet (about 1 g per day).

TABLE 3. Relationship of Drug and Usage Hypertensive Reactions with Various MAOI's. (U.K. Data Only.)

Compound	% Usage[1]	% Reaction known precipitant	% Reaction precipitant unknown
Tranylcypromine	43	70	94
Phenelzine	36	14	2
Isocarboxazid	8	2	—
Nialamide	7	10	—
Others	6	4	4

TABLE 4. Headache Incidence[61] before Cheese Warning was Given and After Warning.

Compound	Before warning		After warning	
	No.	%	No.	%
Tranylcypromine	23/126	18·2	5/119	4·2
Phenelzine	12/259	4·6	2/97	2·0
Isocarboxazid	1/63	1·6	1/28	3·6

(ii) There is a preponderance of cases among the group of monoamine oxidase inhibitors that have a direct amphetamine-like action (e.g. tranylcypromine, phenelzine), although it would appear that all monoamine oxidase inhibitors may produce hypertension when given with appropriate agents. The significance of this relationship can be investigated in three ways:

(a) Table 3 shows the percentage usage of the main monoamine oxidase inhibitors compared with the percentage of reactions with known precipitants and those for no known precipitants. (United Kingdom data throughout.) It will be noted that in both groups tranylcypromine has an incidence that cannot be explained solely on extent of use.

(b) Bethune, Burrell, Culpan and Ogg[61] have undertaken a study of patients in their practice both before the periods when cheese warning was given and after (Table 4). The tranylcypromine preponderance can be seen in the former group. After warnings were given eight cases were seen—in five of these cheese was implicated (the warning had either been omitted or ignored), in two cream, and in one beer.

(c) This difference between monoamine oxidase inhibitors has been further confirmed by the study of headaches reported in papers on iproniazid and isocarboxazid, before the " cheese reaction " was appreciated. In 57 consecutive papers covering 3210 patients who had received isocarboxazid the incidence is 1·8 per cent while in 60 consecutive iproniazid papers on 3274 patients the incidence is 3·2 per cent. This can be compared with tranylcypromine in which the overall incidence is probably over 10 per cent and many series are about 20 per cent.[29, 61, 69, 77]

On the basis of these studies it must be concluded that the incidence is higher with tranylcypromine than other monoamine oxidase inhibitors but giving specific warnings about diet reduces the risks of hypertensive crises from monoamine oxidase inhibitors by 70 per cent or more.

It would appear that the best treatment for the crises is phentolamine.[26, 50, 57, 82]

(3) *Interactions in which an Indirect Action of the Compound Exposes an Unusual Side Effect*

When a compound has a specific biochemical reaction, it is often tempting to ascribe all its effects to this reaction. This has happened in the case of the monoamine oxidase inhibitors. In addition to those causing hypertensive crises, potentiation of other drugs has been described.

(a) *Narcotics.* Potentiation of narcotics has been described by several authors over the past few years,[83–92] and has been ascribed to the monoamine oxidase inhibition.[26, 92, 93]

In fact the potentiation of narcotics has no direct relationship to the monoamine oxidase inhibition. Pethidine, among other compounds is metabolized to a considerable extent by the non-specific oxidase of liver mitochondria.[94] Certain hydrazides among other compounds inhibit these enzymes. There is, however, no relationship between the degree of monoamine oxidase inhibition and that of non-specific oxidase (Table 5). The degree of potentiation due to various monoamine oxidase inhibitors has been studied together with the number of cases attributed to each of the 13 cases where details are available. The lack of correlation is apparent.

(b) *Other compounds.* Non-specific oxidase inhibition by monoamine oxidase inhibitors can cause potentiation of other compounds including barbiturates,[99] phenothiazines[100] and alcohol.[101] This potentiation of alcohol may in part explain some reactions with alcohol after monoamine oxidase inhibitors rather than a tyramine effect.

It is interesting to note that potentiation of both phenothiazines and alcohol has recently been reported from a new cytostatic agent which is a powerful inhibitor of these non-specific oxidases.[102]

(c) *Effect of mebenazine on insulin.* A further indirect effect of a mono-amine oxidase inhibitor, mebenazine, has been described[103]—potentiation of insulin. The presumed mode of action is by interference with catecholamine discharge from storage sites. Further work is necessary before the possibility of other drugs of this class having similar effects[104] can be excluded.

TABLE 5. Relationship of MAOI Activity and Narcotic Potentiation.

Compound	MAOI* activity (mouse)	Narcotic potentiation (mouse)	Number of cases of narcotic potentiation
Iproniazid	1	+++†	5
Isocarboxazid	7	0 ‡	0
Phenelzine	12	+++‡	5
Nialamide	2	—	0
Tranylcypromine	0·6	—	1
Pargyline	2	+++†	2

* MAOI activity as measure *in vivo* by increase of brain 5HT in mice.[95]

† Parkes[96].

‡ Data adapted from. refs. 97-98

REFERENCES

1. Data adapted from usage estimates Intercontinental Medical Services.
2. SIPPEL, W. H., *Rocky. Mtn. med. J.* **55**, 60 (1958).
3. AMIAS, A. G. and FAIRBAIRN, D., *Brit. med. J.* ii, 432 (1963).
4. WAGHMARAE, D., *Brit. med. J.* ii, 936 (1963).
5. MacVICAR, J., *Brit. med. J.* ii, 999 (1963).
6. DONALDSON, I. A., *Brit. med. J.* ii, 1592 (1963).
7. KOPMANN, E. and HUGHES, F. W., *Arch. gen. Psychiat.* **1**, 7 (1959).
8. ZIRKLE, G. A., KING, P. D., McATEE, O. B. and VAN DYKE, R., *J. Amer. med. Ass.* **171**, 1496 (1959).
9. ZIRKLE, G. A., KING, P. D., McATEE, O. B. and VAN DYKE, R., *J. Amer. med. Ass.* **173**, 1823 (1960).
10. GOLDBERG, L., *Quart. J. Stud. Alcohol* Suppl. **1**, 37 (1961).
11. TUTEUR, W. and LEPSEN, D., In *Tranquilizing Drugs*, Ed. Himwich, H. E., Washington, D.C., 1955.
12. BURKITT, E. A. and SUTCLIFFE, C. K., *Brit. med. J.* ii, 1648 (1961).
13. PRANGE, A. J., *Amer. J. Psychiat.* **119**, 994 (1963).
14. OGILVIE, C. M., *Quart. J. Med.* **22**, 511 (1953).
15. SCHILDKRAUT, J. L., KLERMAN, G. L., FRIEND, D. G. and GREENBLATT, M., *Ann. N.Y. Acad. Sci.* **107**, 1005 (1963).
16. POLLIN, W., CARDON, P. V. and KETY, S. S., *Science* **133**, 104 (1961).
17. McGEER, P. L., BOULDING, J. E., GIBSON, W. C. and FOULKES, R. G., *J. Amer. med. Ass.* **177**, 665 (1961).
18. BURN, J. H. and RAND, M. J., *J. Physiol.* **144**, 314 (1958).

19. BRODIE, B. B. and COSTA, E., *Monoamines et Système Nerveux Central*, p. 13, Georg, Geneva, 1961.
20. BABIAK, W., *Canad. med. Ass. J.* **85**, 377 (1961).
21. LUBY, E. D. and DOMINO, E. F., *J. Amer. med. Ass.* **177**, 68 (1961).
22. ROBERTSON, D. S., *Canad. med. Ass. J.* **85**, 711 (1961).
23. LEE, F. I., *Brit. med. J.* **i**, 338 (1961).
24. NYMARK, M. and NIELSEN, I. M., *Lancet* **ii**, 524 (1963).
25. ZECK, P., *Med. J. Aust.* **ii**, 607 (1961).
26. DALLY, P. J., *Lancet* **i**, 1235 (1962).
27. MASON, A., *Lancet* **i**, 1073 (1962).
28. LOW-BEER, G. A. and TIDMARSH, D., *Brit. med. J.* **ii**, 683 (1963).
29. COOPER, A. J., MAGNUS, R. V. and ROSE, M. J., *Lancet* **i**, 527 (1964).
30. SHORE, P. A. and BRODIE, B. B., *Proc. Soc. exp. Biol. N.Y.* **94**, 433 (1957).
31. CHESSIN, M., KRAMER, E. R. and SCOTT, C. C., *J. Pharmacol. exp. Ther.* **119**, 453 (1957).
32. VOELKEL, A., *Ann. N.Y. Acad. Sci.* **80**, 680 (1959).
33. SCHERBEL, A. L., *Amer. J. Cardiol.* **6**, 1125 (1960).
34. HARRER, G., *Wien. med. Wschr.* **111**, 551 (1961).
35. VAN ROSSUM, J. M., *Lancet* **i**, 950 (1963).
36. CLEMENT, A. J. and BENAZON, D., *Lancet* **ii**, 197 (1962).
37. BLACKWELL, B., *Lancet* **ii**, 414 (1963).
38. WOMACK, A. M., *Brit. med. J.* **ii**, 366 (1963).
39. FOSTER, A. R., *Lancet* **ii**, 587 (1963).
40. READ, A. E. A. and ARORA, B., *Lancet* **ii**, 587 (1963).
41. BROOKES (Quoted in WOMACK, A. M.), *Lancet* **ii**, 463 (1963).
42. MAAN, S. S., *Lancet* **ii**, 639 (1963).
43. MILLER, R. B., *Brit. med. J.* **ii**, 1593 (1963).
44. CUTHILL, J. M., GRIFFITHS, A. B. and POWELL, D. E. B., *Lancet* **i**, 1077 (1964).
45. LEONARD, J. W., GIFFORD, R. W. and WILLIAMS, G. H., *Lancet* **i**, 883 (1964).
46. SAWLE THOMAS, J. C., *Brit. med. J.* **ii**, 1406 (1963).
47. EHRLICH, F. and LANGE, F., *Bioch. Z.* **63**, 156 (1914).
48. KOSIKOWSKY, F. V. and DAHLBERG, A. C., *J. Dairy Sci.* **31**, 293 (1948).
49. ASATOOR, A. M., LEVI, A. J. and MILNE, M. D., *Lancet* **ii**, 733 (1963).
50. HORWITZ, D., LOVENBERG, W., ENGELMAN, K. and SJOERDSMA, A., *J. Amer. med. Ass.* **188**, 1108 (1964).
51. UDENFRIEND, S., LOVENBERG, W. and SJOERDSMA, A., *Arch. Biochem.* **85**, 487 (1959).
52. BLACKWELL, B. and MARLEY, E., *Lancet* **i**, 530 (1964).
53. NATOFF, I. L., *Lancet* **i**, 532 (1964).
54. BLACKWELL, B., *Lancet* **ii**, 849 (1963).
55. BLACKWELL, B., MARLEY, E. and RYLE, A., *Lancet* **i**, 722 (1964).
56. HARPER, M., *Lancet* **ii**, 312 (1964).
57. HODGE, J. V., NYE, E. R. and EMERSON, G. W., *Lancet* **i**, 1108 (1964).
58. GUGGENHEIM, M., *Hoppe-Seylers Z. physiol. Chem.* **2**, 88, 276 (1963).
59. IMLAH, N. W., *Med. Wld.* **95**, 187 (1961).
60. DAVIES, E. B., *Lancet* **ii**, 691 (1963).
61. BETHUNE, H. C., BURRELL, R. H., CULPAN, R. H. and OGG, G. J., *Amer. J. Psychiat.* **245**, 121 (1964).
62. MCCLURE, J. L., *Lancet* **i**, 1351 (1962).
63. RAE, J. W. and HARRIMAN, B. P., *Lancet* **i**, 162 (1962).
64. CLARKE, J. A., *Lancet* **i**, 618 (1961).
65. ALDRIGE, M. and OAKLEY, N., *Lancet* **ii**, 932 (1961).
66. BASS, B. H., *Lancet* **ii**, 1099 (1961).
67. DORMER, A. E., *Lancet* **i**, 162 (1962).
68. BLACKWELL, B., *Lancet* **i**, 168 (1963).
69. LEES, F. and BURKE, C. W., *Lancet* **i**, 13 (1963).
70. ENOCH, M. D., *Lancet* **ii**, 464 (1963).
71. MACDONALD, R., *Lancet* **i**, 269 (1963).

72. ARENILLAS, L., *Lancet* **ii**, 586 (1963).
73. GREENE, D., *Lancet* **ii**, 586 (1963).
74. ESPIR, M. L. E. and MITCHELL, L., *Lancet* **ii**, 639 (1963).
75. HURDING, R. F. and MISSEN, H. J., *Brit. med. J.* **ii**, 936 (1963).
76. COOPER, A. J. and ROSE, M. J., *Brit. med. J.* **ii**, 747 (1963).
77. RICHMOND, P. W. and ROBERTS, A. H., *Brit. med. J.* **ii**, 999 (1963).
78. GATES, J. C., *Brit. med. J.* **ii**, 683 (1963).
79. SJOERDSMA, A., LOVENBERG, W., OATES, J. A., CROUT, J. R. and UDENFRIEND, S., *Science* **130**, 225 (1959).
80. COPPEN, A., SHAW, D. M. and FARRELL, J. P., *Lancet* **i**, 79 (1963).
81. PARE, C. M. B., *Lancet* **ii**, 527 (1963).
82. STARK, D. C. C., *Lancet* **i**, 1405 (1962).
83. MITCHELL, R. S., *Ann. int. Med.* **42**, 417 (1955).
84. PAPP, C. and BENAIM, S., *Brit. med. J.* **ii**, 1070 (1958).
85. SHEE, J. C., *Brit. med. J.* **ii**, 507 (1960).
86. PALMER, H., *Brit. med. J.* **ii**, 944 (1960).
87. DENTON, P. H., BORRELLI, V. M. and EDWARDS, N. V., *Brit. med. J.* **ii**, 1752 (1962).
88. TAYLOR, D. C., *Lancet* **ii**, 401 (1962).
89. PELLS COCKS, D. and PASSMORE-ROWE, A., *Brit. med. J.* **ii**, 1545 (1962).
90. REID, N. C. R. W. and JONES, D., *Brit. med. J.* **i**, 408 (1962).
91. BRADLEY, J. J. and FRANCIS, J. G., *Lancet* **i**, 386 (1963).
92. VIGRAN, I. M., *J. Amer. med. Ass.* **187**, 953 (1964).
93. LAWRENCE, D. R., *Prescribers J.* **3**, 46 (1963).
94. LONDON, D. R. and MILNE, M. D., *Brit. med. J.* **ii**, 1752 (1962).
95. ZBINDEN, G., RANDALL, L. O. and MOE, R. A., *Dis. nerv. Syst.* **21**, Sect. 2, 89 (1960).
96. PARKES, M. W., Personal communication.
97. BROWNLEE, G. and WILLIAMS, G. W., *Lancet* **i**, 669 (1963).
98. BROWNLEE, G. and WILLIAMS, G. W., *Lancet* **i**, 1323 (1963).
99. LECHAT, P. and LEMEIGNAN, M., *Biochem. Pharmacol.* **8**, 8 (1961).
100. DEGKWITZ, R. and NESSWETHA, L., *Nervenarzt.* **33**, 138 (1962).
101. SCANLON, W. G., *Ann. N.Y. Acad. Sci.* **80**, 797 (1959).
102. SICHER, C. and BACKHOUSE, T. M., Personal communication.
103. COOPER, A. J. and KEDDIE, K. M. G., *Lancet* **i**, 1133 (1964).
104. VAN PRAAG, H. M. and LEIJNSE, B., *Lancet* **ii**, 103 (1964).

GENERAL DISCUSSION

CHAIRMAN: Dr. Blackwell who with Dr. Marley has done much of the pioneer work on the " cheese reaction " is here and I think it is appropriate if we both congratulate him and invite him to open the general discussion.

B. BLACKWELL (*London*): Thank you, Dr. Sargant. There are some comments I should like to make.

The first thing is, of course, that now that monoamine oxidase inhibitors are used in the treatment of hypertension, as well as in the treatment of depression, the risks of interaction have been considerably increased, and this particularly refers, I think, to alphamethyldopa which is also a hypotensive agent. Furthermore, the people treated with drugs for hypertension are particularly likely to have atherosclerosis or incipient cardiac decompensation which would make the effects of the hypertension much more serious.

Secondly, Bovril, in fact, contains 20 per cent Marmite which may explain why both have this effect. The mode of action of these substances is certainly not tyramine. They do not contain any, and it is probably a histamine-like action very similar to the histamine provocation test one sees in pheochromocytoma.

The third point is that although we warn our patients, they may forget or ignore the warning against eating certain foods and still may suffer from these interactions. I quite agree with Dr. Marks that there will be unexplained cases and also agree that the amino acids in the diet might very well be responsible, after they have been decarboxylated in the gut to form amines. Dr. Marks spoke about clinical reactions with various other precipitating causes and I should like to confirm that these effects can be found in experimental animals not only with tyramine but also with amphetamine, and interestingly enough, the inhibitors themselves, whatever their structure, and also the tricyclic imino dibenzyl derivatives, imipramine and amitriptyline. It also suggests that substances which are neither substrates for amine oxidase nor inhibitors of it may be potentiated after amine oxidase inhibition. This is a puzzle. It is possible, I think, that monoamine oxidase may have yet another function and that many substances form a loose short acting combination with it so that after enzyme inhibition they are capable of releasing noradrenaline from the stores.

Lastly, I cannot agree with some remarks made by Dr. Dally this morning about the personality of people likely to suffer these interactions. I have suffered one myself under experimental conditions. Providing the circumstances and the variables are correct, anybody will suffer from this particular interaction whatever their personality and I think this is to some extent borne out by experimental work in America, and the fact that non-psychiatric patients treated with hypotensive drugs are also quite likely to suffer from these effects.

BERNARD B. BRODIE: Somebody said at an earlier session that desmethylimipramine plus monoamine oxidase was not dangerous when given together. I think this might be so with a very skilled physician. The danger depends upon how completely the monoamine oxidase has been blocked. In animals you can get responses ranging from a mild potentiation to death depending upon the dose of desmethylimipramine and how completely monoamine oxidase has been blocked.

LINFORD REES: I would like to mention the alleged danger of giving amphetamines with monoamine oxidase inhibitors. I think the real danger is when these are given intravenously. The experience of many people in giving amphetamines by mouth with various monoamine oxidase inhibitors is that the reactions are negligible.

F. STEEL (*London*): Using either imipramine or " Parstelin " individually I was only able to obtain, say, 70 to 80 per cent improvement in certain patients. In an effort to step this up to 100 per cent I combined the two drugs and over the years have had perhaps only 20 cases on the combination, but to my knowledge I have had no adverse reactions, though the dosage was small. The results were excellent, but when one or other drug was subsequently discontinued some patients relapsed.

While we must accept that adverse effects have occurred, I think that the combination used discriminately and in small quantities is valuable.

C. M. B. PARE: I would agree that such combinations are useful for the resistant cases but given with care. In particular if the patient is on a monoamine oxidase inhibitor already I introduce the imipramine very slowly indeed. On the other hand, if you give the amine oxidase inhibitor following imipramine, you can give this very much more easily and I would agree with Dr. Sargant with only a small number of side effects.

B. BLACKWELL (*London*): I agree absolutely with what Dr. Pare has said. One wants to differentiate between what happens if you give one drug after another and what happens when you give two drugs together, and it is a situation in which the amine oxidase is completely inhibited and the stores are saturated with catecholamines that is dangerous. If one then introduces another amine there may be trouble.

CHAIRMAN: I think that too much stress has been put on the possible risks of antidepressant drugs. The incidence of such reactions is very small and must be considered in relation to the morbidity and mortality of depression itself, and the acceptable mortality of surgical procedures. If we want to cure our depressions we must take certain calculated risks.

M. HAMILTON: I want to take up further this question of " risks ". Let us not forget that it is the patients who take the risk. The real point, Dr. Sargant, is not that the dangers of these drugs are negligible compared with surgery but that they are avoidable and we must take the necessary precautions, even though they are infrequent.

CHAIRMAN: Does Professor Hamilton think that you must never give iproniazid in case there happens to be a case of infective hepatitis around?

M. HAMILTON: If I knew that there was infective hepatitis around I would seriously consider whether an alternative drug might not be better in the circumstances; and in view of the fact that, for instance, the patients respond well to ECT and do not get liver damage I would probably plump for that.

CHAIRMAN: Would Professor Hamilton ban tranylcypromine because there are 15 deaths in some 4,000,000 people and get say 40 suicides as a result?

M. HAMILTON: I am not suggesting that anything should be banned. I am strongly against those who believe in banning. I am strongly against the practice that is prevalent in America where an administrative authority assumes the right to tell me what I should give or do to my patient. The physician must act as a responsible person.

W. A. H. STEVENSON (*London*): I would like to ask one question. Has there ever been a case in which the vitamin B complex has been implicated when given in large doses? I have had one or two cases of headache which I could not trace to anything in patients on monoamine oxidase inhibitors and vitamin B complex in heavy dosage.

J. MARKS: I know of no cases in the literature. I cannot see theoretically why it should happen.

DRUG THERAPY IN PERSPECTIVE

LINFORD REES

DURING the past two days we have heard of advances in the very complex field of psycho-pharmacology.

Basic research has helped our understanding of the mode of action of various psycho-active drugs. Contributions to our knowledge have come from divergent sources including neurophysiology, biochemistry, pharmacology, animal and human psychology as well as from clinical investigations.

There is a great need for improved methods of assessing clinical status so that the response to drugs can be more scientifically measured. We need data to facilitate more refined methods of selection in order to avoid errors due to heterogeneity of the sample under investigation. Despite these difficulties it seems clear that certain antipsychotic, antidepressive and anti-anxiety drugs do exert significant therapeutically beneficial effects on some patients. It is often found that even when we study apparently clinically homogeneous groups we find that some respond to a particular drug whereas other patients, although clinically similar, derive no benefit.

It seems that we need to know a great deal more about the sub-groups of patients who benefit from particular drugs. It is probable that even when groups are clinically homogeneous they may in fact be heterogeneous in factors which are material to response to drugs; factors such as genetic, constitutional and biochemical attributes. If further research enabled us to select beforehand which patients are likely to respond to specific groups of drugs it would be a major advance and would greatly improve the results obtained by pharmacotherapeutic methods. It is hoped that in the future new drugs will be discovered which have a selective action on the central nervous system and minimal actions on other systems so that side and toxic effects are minimized. We have been reminded that factors other than the pharmacodynamic properties of the drug may influence the results obtained. In this connection social factors and the influence of the therapeutic millieu and other factors may be important and must be taken into account in order to evaluate drug therapy.

Psychiatric illnesses are invariably multi-factorially determined. Social therapy, rehabilitative measures and psychotherapy may be necessary with or without drug therapy to provide effective treatment. To rely on drug therapy alone would be like fighting with one hand behind one's back and the most effective treatment of any illness will be that which is able to modify or influence as many as possible of the relevant and causal factors operating in the particular patient.

Looking back on the past decade we see that many of the important drugs that were responsible for the development of the modern era of psychopharmacology were discovered more by serendipity than by laboratory investigation. Many of the drugs were used empirically but this is not a criticism if the patient derives benefit from the therapy. The history of medicine is full of instances of empirical treatments which were used for many years before their scientific basis became established. There is always a time lag between clinical experience of the effectiveness of a method of treatment and the discovery of its scientific basis.

From the reviews we have heard, it is now evident that there is some scientific basis for drug treatment of psychiatric illness, but this is only the beginning and it is hoped that knowledge will advance with increasing rapidity. For the future we can predict that further progress will be facilitated by greater interdisciplinary co-operation and communication and there appears to be a particularly potentially important role for the clinician who is trained in research and who has the interest and energy to initiate and execute investigations and to collaborate with workers from other scientific fields.

DESIGNATION OF COMPOUNDS AND THEIR CHEMICAL AND TRADE NAMES

DESIGNATIONS, CHEMICAL NOMENCLATURE AND TRADE NAMES OF THE MAIN DRUGS CONSIDERED IN THE SYMPOSIUM

Editors' Note—The left-hand column gives the generic name (or names) where available or the designation used in the text. An effort has been made to give a full list of trade names including both those used in Great Britain and overseas.

Acepromazine	2-acetyl-10-(3-dimethylaminopropyl)-phenothiazine maleate	" Notensil " " Tindal "
Acetoxymethane	laevo isomer of 1-phenyl-1-(2-piperidyl)-1-acetoxymethane hydrochloride	" Supramin "
Amitriptyline	5-(3-dimethylaminopropylidene)-dibenzo [a,d-][1,4] cycloheptadiene hydro- chloride	" Laroxyl " " Tryptizol' " Saroten " " Elavil " (U.S.A.)
		" Benzedrine "
Amphetamine (dexamphetamine)	(±)-α-methylphenethylamine sulphate	
Amylobarbitone	5-ethyl-5-isopentylbarbituric acid	" Amytal "
Amylobarbitone sodium	Mono sodium derivative of 5-ethyl-5-isopentyl barbituric acid	" Sodium Amytal "
" Anxine "	dexamphetamine sulphate	" Anxine "
	mephenesin	
	cyclobarbitone	
Benactyzine	2-diethylaminoethyl benzilate hydrochloride	" Cevanol " " Lucidil " " Suavitil " " Nutinal "
Benzquinamide	N, N-diethyl-1,3,4,6,7,11b hexahydro-2-hydroxy-9,10-dimethoxy-2H-benzo [a] quinolizine-3-carboxamide acetate	" Quantril " (U.S.A.)
Carphenazine	10-[3-(4-[2-hydroxyethyl]-1-piperazinyl)-propyl-2-proprionylphenothiazine bis hydrogen maleate	" Proketazine " (U.S.A.)

Compound	Chemical name	Trade name
Chlorodiazepoxide	7-chloro-2-methylamino-5-phenyl-3H-1,4-benzodiazepine-4-oxide	"Librium"
Chlorpromazine	2-chloro-10-(3-dimethylaminopropyl) phenothiazine hydrochloride	"Largactil"
		"Thorazine" (U.S.A.)
Chlorprothixene	2-chloro-9-(3-dimethylaminopropylidene) thioxanthene	"Taractan"
		"Truxal" (Dan)
Dehydro-iso-androsterone		"Diandrone"
Desipramine Desmethylimipramine	5-(3-methylaminopropyl)-10,11-dihydrodibenz [b, f] azepine	"Pertofran"
Dexamphetamine-Amylobarbitone mixture	(+)-α-methylphenethylamine sulphate mg 5 with amylobarbitone (q.v.) mg 32	"Drinamyl"
Diazepam	7-chloro-1,3-dihydro-1-methyl-5-phenyl-2H-1,4-benzodiazepine-2-one	"Valium"
Dipiperon	1-[3-(p-fluorobenzoyl) propyl]-4-carboxamido-4-piperidino piperidine	"Piperonyl"
Ethyl biscoumacetate	Ethyl Bis (4-hydroxycoumarinyl) acetate	"Tromexan"
Etryptamine	3-(2-aminobutyl) indole acetate	"Monase"
Fluopromazine (Trifluopromazine)	10-(3-dimethylaminopropyl)-2-trifluoromethylphenothiazine hydrochloride	"Vespral"
		"Vesprin" (U.S.A.)
		"Siquil" (abroad)
Fluphenazine	10-[3-(4-[2-hydroxethyl] piperazin-1-yl) propyl]-2-trifluromethylphenothiazine dihydrochloride	"Moditen"
		"Prolixen" (U.S.A.)
		"Permitel" (U.S.A.)
Guanethidine	N-[2-(octahydro-1-azocinyl) ethyl] guanidine sulphate	"Ismelin"
Haloanisone	1-[3-(p-fluorobenzoyl) propyl]-4-(2-methoxyphenyl) piperazine	
Haloperidol	4-(4-chlorophenyl)-1-[3-(4-fluorobenzoyl) propyl]-piperidin-4-ol	"Serenace"
Imipramine	5-(3-dimethylaminopropyl)-10,11-dihydrodibenz [b, f] azepine hydrochloride	"Tofranil"
Iproniazid	N-isonicotinoyl-N^1-isopropylhydrazine phosphate	"Marsilid"
Isocarboxazid	3-N^1-benzylhydrazinocarbonyl-5 methylisoxazole	"Marplan"
Isoniazid	isonicotinoyl hydrazine	"Rimifon"
		"Cotinazin"
		"I.N.H."
		"Mybasan"
		"Neumandin"
		"Nicetal"

Compound	Chemical name	Trade name(s)
		"Nydrazid"
		"Pycazide"
		"Tubomel"
		"Vazadrine"
Mebanazine	α-methylbenzyl hydrozine	"Actomol"
Mephenesin	3-(2-methylphenoxy) propone-1,2-diol	"Myanesin"
		"Tolseram"
		"Lissephen"
Meprobamate	2,2-di(carbamoyloxymethyl) pentane	"Equanil"
		"Miltown"
		"Mepavlon"
Methamphetamine	d-N, -α-dimethylphenethylamine hydrochloride	"Methedrine"
Methotrimeprazine (laevomepromazine)	(−)-10-(3-dimethylamino-2-methylpropyl)-2-methoxyphenothiazine acid maleate or hydrochloride	"Veractil" "Nozinan" (Fr.)
Methoxypromazine	10-(3-dimethylaminopropyl)-2-methoxy-phenothiazine maleate	"Tentone" (U.S.A.)
Methylpentynol	3-methylpent-1-yn-3-ol	"Oblivon" "Somnesin"
Nialamide	N-(2-benzylcarbamoylethyl)-N^1-isonicotinoylhydrazine	"Niamid"
Norethandrolone	17α-ethyl-19-nortestosterone	"Nilevar"
Nortriptyline	5-(3-methylaminopropylidene)-dibenzo [a,d][1,4] cyclohepta-diene hydrochloride	"Aventyl" "Allegron"
Opipranol	5-[3-(4-hydroxyethylpiperazin-1-yl) propyl] dibenz [b, f] azepine	"Insidon"
Orphenadrine	2-dimethylaminoethyl 2-methyldiphenyl-methyl ether hydrochloride	"Disipal"
Oxymetholone	17β-hydroxy-2-hydroxymethylene-17α-methyl-5α-androstan-3-one	"Anapolon" "Adroyd"
Oxypertine	1-[2-(5, 6-dimethoxy-2-methyl-3-indolyl) ethyl]-4-phehylpiperazine	"Eutonyl"
Pargyline	N-benzyl-N-methyl-propargylamine	—
Pecazine (Mepazine)	10-(1-methyl-3-piperidylmethyl) phenothiazine hydrochloride or acetate	"Pacatal"
Pentobarbitone sodium	Mono sodium derivative of 5-ethyl-5-(1-methylbutyl) barbituric acid	"Nembutal"
Perphenazine	2-chloro-10-(3-[4-(2-hydroxyethyl) piperazin-1-yl]-propyl) phenothiazine	"Fentazin" "Trilafon" (U.S.A.)
Phenelzine	phenethylhydrazine hydrogen sulphate	"Nardil"
Pheniprazine	α-methylphenethylhydrazine hydrochloride	"Cavodil" "Catron" (U.S.A.)

Phenobarbitone	5-ethyl-5-phenylbarbituric acid	"Luminal" "Gardenal"
Phenoxypropazine	(1-methyl-2-phenoxyethyl) hydrazine hydrogen maleate	"Drazine"
Piperacetazine	2-acetyl-10-(3-[4-(2-hydroxyethyl) piperidino]-propyl) phenothiazine	"Quide" (U.S.A.)
Prochlorperazine	2-chloro-10-[3-(4-methylpiperazin-1-yl) propyl] phenothiazine dimaleate	"Stemetil" "Compazine" (U.S.A.)
Promazine	10-(3-dimethylaminopropyl) phenothiazine hydrochloride	"Sparine"
Promethazine	10-(2-dimethylaminopropyl) phenothiazine hydrochloride	("Verophen") "Phenergan"
Reserpine	Alkaloid from *Rauwolfia* spp.	"Serpasil"
"Sedaltine"	carbromal bromvaletone aluminium hydroxide *Rauwolfia* mephenesin	"Sedaltine"
Stilboestrol	3,4-di(4-hydroxyphenyl) hex-3-ene	
Tetrabenazine	1,2,3,4,6,7-hexahydro-3-isobutyl-9,10-dimethoxybenzo-[a] quinolizin-2-one	"Nitoman"
Thiopropazate	10-(3-[4-(2-acetoxyethyl) piperazin-1-yl] propyl)-2-chlorophenothiazine hydrochloride	"Dartalan"
Thioproperazine	2-dimethylsulphamoyl-10-(3-(4-methylpiperazin-1-yl)-propyl phenothiazine mesylate	"Majeptil"
Thioridazine	10-[2-(1-methyl-2-piperidyl) ethyl]-2-methylthiophenothiazine hydrochloride	"Melleril"
Tranylcypromine	(±)-*trans*-2-phenylcyclopropylamine sulphate	"Parnate"
Trifluoperazine	10-[3-(4-methylpiperazin-1-yl) propyl]-2-trifluoromethylphenothiazine dihydrochloride	"Stelazine" ("Terfluzin")
Trifluoperidol (Triperidol)	1-[3-(*p*-fluorobenzoyl) propyl]-4-hydroxy-4-(3-trifluoromethylphenyl) piperidine	

INDEX

Acetophenazine 15
Acetoxymethane 83
"Actomol"—*see* Mebanazine
Adenosine diphosphate 153
" Adroyd "—*see* Oxymetholone
Alcohol
  alcoholism 180
  potentiation of 193, 196, 198
" Allegron "—*see* Nortriptyline
Alpha methyldopa 195, 202
Amitriptyline
  clinical use of 149, 185
  drug interactions of 193, 194, 202
  effect on platelet serotonin 148
  mode of action of 143
Amphetamine
  clinical use of 83
  difference of effect in children 150
  drug interactions of 194, 202
  effects on animals 35, 134
  metabolism 95
  persistence of effect of 47
  potentiation of, with disipramine 139
Amygdala
  anatomy of 10
  effect of
    chlordiazepoxide 19
    extirpation 11
  physiological role of 11
Amylobarbitone 80
  ataxia in animals 32
  effect of, in stressed rats 26
  stimulant effects in rats of 29
  use in anxiety states 159, 180
Amylobarbitone sodium 57
" Amytal "—*see* Amylobarbitone
" Anapolon "—*see* Oxymetholone
Anticonvulsant tests 168
Antidepressants
  classification of 103
  clinical use of 103 et seq., 149
  effect of on EEG 16
  general description of 16
  selection of 107–110
  sites of action—summary 22
Anxiety states
  drug treatment of 157 et seq., 179–181, 185

mode of action of anti-anxiety drugs in 165 et seq.
problems of definition of 181
relation to depression 150, 157, 181, 182, 185, 186
use of
  barbiturates in 159, 179
  meprobamate in 161, 179, 187
  phenothiazines in 57, 160, 179
" Anxine " 179
Ascorbic acid—in schizophrenia 83
ATP—*see* " High energy " phosphate esters
ATP-ase, inhibition by chlorpromazine 65
" Aventyl "—*see* Nortriptyline

Barbiturates—*see also* under separate members of the group
  effect of, on
    body temperature 51
    reticular formation 20
  effect of temperature on results 51
  potentiation of 198
  sites of action—summary 22
  stimulant effects of 29
  undesirable characteristics of 21, 159
  use in anxiety states 159
Benactyzine
  effect of, in experimental neuroses 28
  in anxiety states 179
" Benzedrine "—*see* Amphetamine
Benzoquinolizines—*see also* Tetrabenazine, Benzquinamide and Ro 4–1284
  action of, on catecholamines 123
  clinical use of 84
  side effects of 84
Benzquinamide 84, 139
Betaine—in schizophrenia 90, 92
Body temperature
  effect of, on
    behaviour 35, 51
    phenothiazine results in animals 96, 197
" Bovril " 196, 202
Brain
  amines 119, 152
  centre for emotional behaviour co-ordination 5

211

P

Brain (*cont.*)
  phosphates—*see* " High energy " phosphate esters
  phospholipids 66
  reverberating circuit concept 4
  tissue respiration with phenothiazines 65
Brain hexokinase
  effect of methamphetamine on 50
  in schizophrenia 50
Broad beans 196
Butyrophenones 84
  see also under names of individual drugs

Carphenazine 15
Catecholamine—*see also* under noradrenaline and adrenaline
  agglutination of platelets 153
  effect of
    DMI on 136, 153
    phenothiazines on transport of, across membranes 68, 96, 97, 153
    imipramine 152
  in hypertensive crises 194
  pool theory 117
Catechol-*O*-methyl-transferase 117
" Catron "—*see* Pheniprazine
" Cavodil "—*see* Pheniprazine
" Cevanol "—*see* Benactyzine
Cheese 195
Children, psychiatric disorders of
  anxiety states in 186
  depressions in 149
  use of phenothiazines in 58
Chlordiazepoxide
  combined with other drugs, 150, 162
  effect of, in limbic structures 19
  mode of action of 167 et seq.
  side effects of 163
  sites of action—summary 22
  use of in
    alcoholism 180
    anxiety states 162, 180, 185
    depressive states 162
    obsessive compulsive syndrome 162
    schizophrenia 80
Chlorpromazine
  clinical use of 57, 58, 59, 61
  effect of, in
    anxiety states 160, 179
  effect of, on
    body weight of disturbed rats 36
    brain amines 96
    platelets 148, 152, 153
  mode of action 64 et seq.
  structure functional relationship 75, 76

Chlorprothixene 160
Clinical trials 95, 148, 205
  see also under Controlled and Uncontrolled trials
Cocaine 195
  effects of in platelets 148, 153
" Compazine "—*see* Prochlorperazine
Conditioned avoidance
  effect of
    anti-anxiety compounds on 168 et seq.
    phenothiazine on 28, 175
    reserpine on 28
Controlled trials 39, 56, 141, 160, 185
  assessment of psychological changes in 41, 51, 52
  inferences based on patient selection 40
  selection of patients for 40
  statistical handling of score data in 42
  suggested design for comparison of drugs in 77
Cortex, cerebral—effect of anti-anxiety drugs on 177
Corticotrophin—in schizophrenia 81
Cortisone—in schizophrenia 81
Creatine phosphate—*see* " High energy " phosphate esters
Cytochrome oxidase—inhibition of, by chlorpromazine 65

" Dartalan "—*see* Thiopropazate
Decarboxylase 154
Degenerative brain lesions—influencing reactions to phenothiazines 61, 187
Dehydro-iso-androsterone—in schizophrenia 81, 96
Demethylation
  of amines affecting their activity 143, 153
  of phenothiazines 97, 153
Depressive states
  relationship to, to anxiety states 150, 158, 181, 182, 185, 186
  similarity of, to reserpine effects 129
  therapy 103 et seq.
  use of
    chlordiazepoxide in 162
    phenothiazine in 58, 96–98
Desdimethylimipramine 148
Desipramine (DMI)
  an active form of imipramine 132 et seq.
  danger in combinations 202
  effect of, on
    platelet serotonin 148
    rats of different strains and ages 140

effect of, with benzoquinolizines 133, 141
mechanism of action of 136, 145, 153
metabolism 136, 141
properties of 132
species differences in response 140
Desmethyl chlorpromazine 153
Desmethylimipramine—see Desipramine
Desmethylpromazine 143
Desmethyltrifluopromazine 143
Dexamphetamine—see Amphetamine
Dexamphetamine–amylobarbitone mixture
    ataxia on 31
    effects of, in animals 30, 152
    persistence of effects 47
    potentiation of effects 31
Diamine oxidase 154
" Diandrone "—see Dehydro-iso-andro-
    sterone
Diazepam
    mode of action of 167
    side effects of 163
    use of, in
        anxiety states 162, 180
        schizophrenia 80
Diazepines—see also under individual
    compounds
    mode of action of 167 et seq.
    side effects of 163
    use of, in anxiety states 161
Dicoumarol 142
Differences between results of treatment in
    normals and patients 50–52
3,4-dihydroxyphenylalanine—see DOPA
Dimethoxyphenylethylamine—isolation
    from schizophrenics 90
Dipiperon 88
Discontinuous treatment of schizophrenia
    60
" Disipal "—see Orphenadrine
DOPA
    as precursor of catecholamines 120, 124
    drug interactions 194, 196
    potentiation of, by desipramine 140
Dopamine
    effect of monoamine oxidase inhibitors
        119
    sites of high concentration of 12
" Drazine "—see Phenoxypropazine
Dreaming 187
" Drinamyl "—see Dexamphetamine–amy-
    lobarbitone mixture
Drug combinations
    amitriptyline and phenothiazines 83
    extent of use 192
    imipramine and chlordiazepoxide 162
    imipramine and " Parstelin " 203
    imipramine and phenothiazines 150

monoamine oxidase inhibitors and ami-
    triptyline 150, 185
monoamine oxidase inhibitors and
    amphetamine 202
monoamine oxidase inhibitors and
    chlordiazepoxide 150, 162
monoamine oxidase inhibitors and
    imipramine 150, 202
side effects of 191 et seq., 202
Drug interactions 191 et seq.
    see also " Combinations of drugs "

EEG
    association of affect with arousal re-
        action 9
    effect of
        anti-anxiety drugs on 177
        antidepressants on 16
        phenothiazines on 74, 96, 177
    reticular formation in arousal reaction of
        8
" Elavil "—see Amitriptyline
Electro-convulsive therapy
    clinical use of 58, 147, 151, 185
    problems of 61, 112
Environment
    effect of, in
        animals on drug studies 36, 45, 51
        humans on drug studies 44
Enzyme systems
    effect of
        chlorpromazine on 65
        monoamine oxidase inhibitors on
            116, 154, 198
" Equanil "—see Meprobamate
Ethyl biscoumacetate 142
Etryptamine 112
" Eutonyl "—see Pargyline
Experimental neuroses 28
Extent of usage of
    antidepressants 112
    monoamine oxidase inhibitors 197
    psychotropic drugs 50
Extrapyramidal systems 143, 193
    persistent 61, 187
    therapy of 143
    with phenothiazine 57–60

" Fentazin "—see Perphenazine
Flavoprotein antagonism—by phenothi-
    azine 65
Fluopromazine 14
Fluphenazine 15
Food intake tests 168
Frontal lobe orbital surface
    effect of extirpation of 11
    physiological role of 11

Ganglion blocking drugs 193
" Gardenal "—see Phenobarbitone
Genetic aspects 51, 205
  in response to antidepressants 107, 152
Glycocyamine 91
Guanethidine 315

Hallucinations—effect of phenothiazine on
  57
Hallucinogens 90
Haloanisone 88
Haloperidol 58, 85, 96
Headaches—see also Hypertensive crises
  with monoamine oxidase inhibitors 151,
  202
" High energy " phosphate ester—effect of
  chlorpromazine on 65, 66
Hippocampus
  anatomy of 10
  effect of
    chlordiazepoxide on 19
    meprobamate on 20
2-hydroxydesmethylimipramine 148
5-hydroxytryptamine
  brain levels of under treatment in humans
    106
  effect of
    monoamine oxidase inhibitors 119
    phenothiazines upon membrane trans-
      fer of 68
    reserpine 13
  in human thrombocytes 119, 147, 152
  sites of high concentration of 11
Hypertensive crises with monoamine oxidase inhibitors 151, 194 et seq.
Hypertensives—drugs potentiation 193,
  202
Hypothalamus
  effect of
    anti-anxiety drugs on 177
    barbiturates on 21
    reserpine on 14
  physiological importance of 5

Imipramine
  antagonism of reserpine effects 130
  clinical use of 83, 106, 149, 152
  drug interactions of 193, 194, 203
  effects in thrombocytes 148, 152, 153
  mode of action of 128 et seq.
  species differences in response to 141
  time response study 130
Imipramine-like antidepressants—see Thymoleptics

" Insidon "—see Opipranol
Insulin—in schizophrenia 81
Iproniazid
  actions of on enzymes 125, 154
  biochemical effects of 120
  chemical structure of 116
  clinical use of 105, 110, 150, 185
  hypertensive crises with 194, 198
  incidence of jaundice with 112
  releasing monoamines 123
" Ismelin "—see Guanethidine
Isocarboxazid
  chemical structure of 116
  clinical use of 83, 106, 110, 150, 185
  incidence of
    hypertensive crises with 198
    jaundice with 112
Isoniazid 125

Laevomepromazine—see Methotrimepra-
  zine
" Largactil "—see Chlorpromazine
" Laroxyl "—see Amitriptyline
Learning—effect of drugs on, in animals 34
Leucotomy 150, 185
" Librium "—see Chlordiazepoxide
Limbic system
  anatomy and interconnections of 5, 9–
    11
  effect of
    anti-anxiety drugs on 177
    barbiturates on 21
    chlordiazepoxide on 19
    meprobamate on 20
    reserpine on 14
  physiological role of different parts of 11
  results of extirpations of 11
Lithium carbonate 58, 152
" Lissephen "—see Mephanesin
" Lucidil "—see Benactyzine
" Luminal "—see Phenobarbitone

" Majeptil "—see Thioproperazine
Mania
  effect of phenothiazine on 58
  treatment of, with
    imipramine 152
    lithium 152
" Marmite " 196, 202
" Marplan "—see Isocarboxazid
" Marsilid "—see Iproniazid
Mebanazine 110, 199
" Melleril "—see Thioridazine
" Mepavlon "—see Meprobamate
Mepazine—see Pecazine
Mephanesin 179

Meprobamate
  effect of, on limbic system 19
  mode of action of 167
  sites of action of—summary 22
  use of, in
    anxiety states 161, 179
    schizophrenia 80
Mescaline 90
  persistence of effects of 50
Mesodiencephalic activating system
  effect of
    barbiturates on 20
    phenothiazines on 15
  physiology of 8
Metabolism—of phenothiazines 66
Methamphetamine
  effect of, on brain hexokinase 50
  persistence of effect of 50
" Methedrine "—see Methamphetamine
Methionine—in schizophrenia 90, 92
Methotrimeprazine 58, 59, 98
Methoxypromazine 14
Methylpentynol 179
α methyl m-tyrosine 136
Miller's experiments on rats 26, 51, 52
" Miltown "—see Meprobamate
Mode of actions—see also under separate
    drug classes
  summary 22
" Moditen "—see Fluphenazine
Monoamine oxidase inhibitors—see also
    under separate drug names
  biochemical differences related to res-
    ponse 109
  clinical use of 105 et seq., 149, 185, 186
  general description of 16
  hypertensive crises with 151, 193 et seq.,
    202
  in schizophrenia 83
  pharmacology of 116 et seq.
  potentiation of other drugs by 154,
    193 et seq., 202
  sites of action—summary 22
" Monase "—see Etryptamine
Motor restlessness—use of phenothiazine
    58
Muscle relaxation 168
" Myanesin "—see Mephenesin

Narcotics 198
" Nardil "—see Phenelzine
" Nembutal "—see Pentobarbitone-sodium
Nialamide 110, 116, 120
" Niamid "—see Nialamide
Nicotinamide—in schizophrenia 83, 91
Nicotinic acid—in schizophrenia 83, 91

" Nilevar "—see Norethandrolone
" Nitoman "—see Tetrabenazine
N-methyl adrenaline 91
Non specific oxidase 154, 198
Noradrenaline
  effect of
    imipramine on 153
    reserpine on 13
  metabolism 117
  sites of high concentration of 11
  transport across membranes—effect of
    phenothiazines on 67
Norepinephrine—see Noradrenaline
Norethandralone 81
Normetadrenaline 119
Nortriptyline 143, 144, 148
" Nozinan "—see Methotrimeprazine
" Nutinal "—see Benactyzine

" Oblivon "—see Methylpentynol
Obsessive compulsive syndrome—use of
    chlordiazepoxide in 162, 187
Oestrogens—in schizophrenia 82
Operant conditioning experiments 168
    et seq.
Opipranol 16
Orphenadrine 61, 83, 148
Oxymetholone—in schizophrenia 82
Oxypertine 84

" Pacatal "—see Pecazine
Papez circuit 5
Pargyline 116, 125
Parkinsonism—see Extrapyramidal symp-
    toms
" Parnate "—see Tranylcypromine
Pecazine 14, 75–76
Pentobarbitone sodium
  differing effects of, in human experiments
    26
  use in anxiety states 159
Perception—effects of drugs on 33
" Permitel "—see Fluphenazine
Perphenazine 15, 59, 61
  use of, in
    anxiety states 160, 180
    depression 97
Persistence of effects after drug discontinu-
    ation
  in animals 32
  in humans 47, 50
" Pertofran "—see Desipramine
Pethidine 193, 198

Phenelzine
  chemical structure of 116
  clinical use of 110, 150, 185
  hypertensive crises with 197
" Phenergan "—see Promethazine
Pheniprazine 112, 116
Phenobarbitone
  mode of action 167 et seq.
  stimulant effect of, in animals 29
  use in anxiety states 159
Phenothiazines—see also individual compounds
  clinical use of 55 et seq., 179
  effect of, in
    conditioned avoidance experiments 25
    depression 97, 98
  effect of, on
    body temperature 51
    neocortical areas 15
  inhibition of transport across membranes by 67, 96, 153
  metabolism of 66
  mode of action 63 et seq., 97
  pharmacological effects of, in mid brain 14
  side effects of 58 et seq., 76, 187
  sites of action of—summary 22
Phenoxypropazine 150
Phentolamine 198
Phenylalanine 196, 202
Phobic states—relation to anxiety 182, 186
Piperacetazine 14
" Piperonyl "—see Dipiperon
Pituitary-adrenal system—effect of phenothiazines on 66
Plasma corticosteroids—effect of chlorpromazine 66
Platelets—see Thrombocytes
Prochlorperazine 14
  chemical structure of 75
  clinical use of 58–59
" Proketazine "—see Carphenazine
" Prolixen "—see Fluphenazine
Promazine 14
  clinical use of 58, 160
  structure activity relationship of 75, 76
Promethazine 58, 61, 72
Psychological changes
  assessment in patients 41, 50, 51
  relevance of some changes 45
Psychotherapeutic aspects 93, 183, 186, 187, 205

" Quantril "—see Benzquinamide
" Quide "—see Piperacetazine

Rating scales 41
Rauwolfia alkaloid—see also Reserpine
  effect on catecholamines 123, 194
Relevance of animal experiments to human activity 28, 50, 186
Reserpine
  clinical use of 57, 84
  effect of, on
    conditioned avoidance experiments 25
    hypothalamic mechanisms 13
    limbic structures 14
    neurohormones 13, 124, 129, 193–194
  inducing sleep pattern 13
  preliminary effect of, on reticular formation 13
  sites of action—summary 22
Reticular formation
  anatomy of 8 et seq.
  effect of
    anti-anxiety drugs on 177
    barbiturates on 20
    phenothiazines on 74
    reserpine on 13
  in EEG arousal reaction 8
Ro 4–1284 132
Ro 4–4602 124, 125
Ro 4–5360 47

" Saroten "—see Amitriptyline
Schizophrenia
  abnormal sensitivities in 61
  discontinuous treatment—phenothiazine 60
  levels of brain hexokinase in 50
  methylation in 90
  possible future trends in treatment 90 et seq.
  treatment of, other than phenothiazines 79 et seq.
  use of phenothiazines in 57 et seq.
" Sedaltine " 179
Sedative action of
  phenothiazines 57
  Ro 4–5360 48
Septal area
  effect of
    chlordiazepoxide on 19
    extirpation 11
    physiological role of 11
" Serenace "—see Haloperidol
Serotonin—see 5 hydroxytryptamine
" Serpasil "—see Reserpine
Side effects—see also under separate compounds of
  barbiturates 159
  butyrophenones 85

diazepines   163
drug combinations   191 et seq.
meprobamate   162
monoamine oxidase inhibitors   110
oxypertine   84
phenothiazines   58 et seq., 76, 187
reserpine and related drugs   84
" Siquil "—see Fluopromazine
Social aspects—influencing results   60, 93
    et seq., 97–98, 205
" Sodium amytal "—see Amylobarbitone
    sodium
" Somnesin "—see Methylpentynol
" Sparine "—see Promazine
" Stelazine "—see Trifluoperazine
" Stemetil "—see Prochlorperazine
Stilboestrol—in schizophrenia   82
Stressed animal studies—effect of amylo-
    barbitone   26
Structure function relationships   58, 71 et
    seq., 143
" Suavityl "—see Benactyzine
Subjective experience—interpretation from
    animal results   50–51
" Supramin "—see Acetoxymethane

Taming effects   167
" Taractan "—see Chlorprothixene
" Tentone "—see Methoxypromazine
" Terfluzin "—see Trifluoperazine
Tetrabenazine   84, 141
Thalamus—effect of anti-anxiety drugs on
    177
Thiamine oxidase   154
Thiopropazate   59, 96, 98
Thioproperazine—in schizophrenia   59–61
Thioridazine
    chemical structure of   75
    clinical use of   59–60, 160
" Thorazine "—see Chlorpromazine
Thrombocytes—monoamine   changes   in
    119, 147, 152
Thymoleptics—see   also   under   separate
    names of drugs
    general description of   16
    mode of action of   124, 128 et seq.
    sites of action—summary   22

Thyroid
    drug interaction involving   193
    in schizophrenia   80, 96
" Tindal "—see Acepromazine
" Tofranil "—see Imipramine
" Tolseram "—see Mephenesin
Toxic effects, of antidepressants   112
Tranylcypromine
    chemical structure of   116
    clinical use of   150
    enzyme activity   125
    hypertensive reactions   196, 203
    possible   direct   sympathomimetic   action
    125, 197
Trifluoperazine   15
    clinical use of   59–60, 83–84, 160
    structure functional relationships of   75
    76
Trifluoperidol   86 et seq.
Triflupromazine—see Fluopromazine
" Trilafon "—see Perphenazine
Triperidol—see Trifluoperidol
" Tromexan "—see Ethylbiscoumacetate
" Truxal "—see Chlorprothixene
Tryptophan
    in man   111, 124, 197
    interaction   with   monoamine   oxidase
    110–111, 120
" Tryptizol "—see Amitriptyline
Tyramine   202
    effect on thrombocyte serotonin   152
    in cheese   195
Tyrosine   196, 202

Uncontrolled   clinical   trials—problems   of
    assessment   40

" Valium "—see Diazepam
Variability in reaction to drugs   34–36
" Veractil "—see Methotrimeprazine
" Verophen "—see Promazine
" Vespral "—see Fluopromazine
" Vesprin "—see Fluopromazine
Vitamin B complex   203